Medical Parasitology: Practical Exercises and Principles

Mukhlisa Turopova

Medical Parasitology: Practical Exercises and Principles

by: Mukhlisa Turopova

Edition: December '2025
Publisher:
Taemeer Publications LLC (Michigan, USA / Hyderabad, India)

ISBN 978-93-6908-396-1

Book	:	**Medical Parasitology: Practical Exercises and Principles**
Author	:	Mukhlisa Turopova
Publisher	:	Taemeer Publications
Year	:	'2025
Pages	:	188
Title Design	:	*Taemeer Web Design*

INTRODUCTION

In recent years, the science of parasitology has become an integral part of various sectors of the national economy, as well as important problems such as environmental protection. Its fields, especially medical parasitology, veterinary parasitology, and phytoparasitology, are developing rapidly.

Some brief information about parasitic organisms is given to undergraduate biology students in the first year of the course of invertebrate zoology. However, this brief information is not enough for students. Teaching Parasitology based on practical exercises helps to further consolidate and expand the knowledge gained by students in zoology.

This educational methodical guide provides necessary information on the systematic status of common parasites, their morphological and anatomical structure, and development cycle, which are mainly found in humans and productive animals in our republic and cause various parasitic diseases. The educational methodical guide also provides necessary advice on the materials and equipment needed by students to complete each practical exercise, as well as the procedure for conducting the exercise.

1-PRACTICAL TRAINING

Subject: Parasite one from cells - the structure and development of amoeba, trypanosomes, and leishmania

Case 1. The structure and development cycle of amoeba enterica

Systematic status of intestinal amoeba

Small world. Unicellular animals – Protozoa

Type. Sarcomastigophora - Sarcomastigophora

Junior type. Sarcodina - Sarcodina

Class: Rhizopoda

Category. Amoebae - Amoebina

Representative. Enteric amoeba - Entamoeba histolytica

Required materials and equipment: Stained micropreparations of amoeba enterica, overhead projector, microscope, color tables depicting the structure and development cycle of amoeba enterica.

Objective: To study the structure, development cycle, distribution, and harm of the intestinal amoeba, a parasite that infects humans.

Brief content of the topic. The species that live parasitically within the class of the amoebae mainly belong to the order of amoebae. Several species of the order of amoebae are parasitic in humans and animals. Among them, the dysentery amoeba parasitizes in the large intestine of humans and causes amoebiasis, that is, bloody diarrhea. In general, 5 species of amoebae are found in the human body. Four of them are considered harmless and live mainly as bacteria in the colon and cecum.

Amoeba enterica was first identified in 1875 by the Russian physician A.F. Lesh, who proved that this amoeba is pathogenic (harmful). The size of the amoeba enterica is 20-30 microns.

During the development of amoeba enterica, cystic and vegetative forms occur. The vegetative form, in turn, is divided into small vegetative, tissue, and hematophagous or erythrophagous forms (Fig. 1).

The tissue and erythrophagous forms of amoeba are sometimes called the large vegetative form. In fact, these two forms differ in their habitat and method of feeding. The cyst is usually round in shape and is surrounded by a dense membrane - the cyst shell.

A mature cyst has 4 nuclei, and an immature one has 1-2. The vegetative form is small and motile. Its cytoplasm is sharply divided into two - a clear, translucent ectoplasm and a granular endoplasm. A spherical nucleus is located in the endoplasm. The vegetative form lives in the large intestine of a person, feeds on bacteria, and does not cause harm to humans. The dysentery amoeba lives in the walls of the human large intestine, creating ulcers and feeding by eating away at the tissues in the intestinal wall.

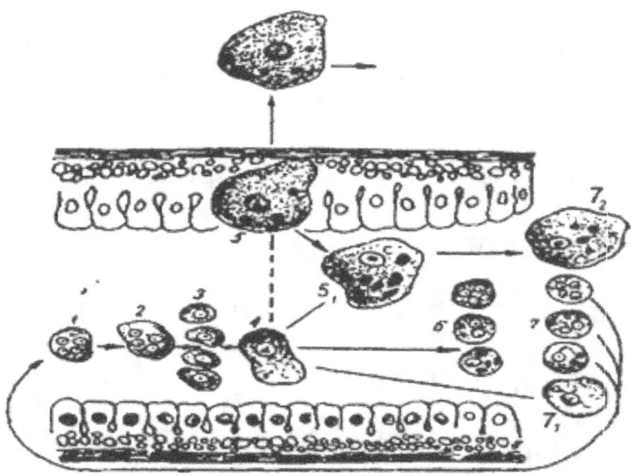

1st cm . The scheme of the development cycle of Entamoeba histolytica :

1st grade road system ; 2- the work of the system of a myob a ; The 3-4th cavity is closed v e g e t a tive sh a kll a ri; 5th large vegetative sh a kli ; 6th internal system ; 7 - thousands of slimy waste The shape of the three .

The small vegetative form of amoeba enterica is considered the main form. Because it multiplies into tissue forms - erythrophages and cysts. Cysts are resistant to the external environment and do not die even in chlorinated water. Lung injury occurs when a liver abscess passes through the diaphragm into the lungs. The main symptoms of amebiasis are abdominal pain, loss of appetite, diarrhea with pus and blood. To diagnose the disease, the patient's feces are collected in a preservative and examined. The composition of the preservative was proposed by A.A. Turdiyev in 1971.

Procedure. Stain a preparation obtained from the bloody mucus of a person suffering from amoebic dysentery in iron hemotoxin according to the Heidenhain method and examine it under a microscope. When you examine the preparation, you will see erythrocytes, which are stained black. Amoebic dysentery is visible among the erythrocytes.

Look at the preparation of intestinal amoeba under a microscope. In terms of size, intestinal amoeba is similar to dysentery amoeba. There are many vacuoles in its protoplasm. A large, spongy nucleus is visible inside it. Upon careful examination, bacteria and starch grains can be seen in the vacuoles. The cysts of intestinal amoeba are round. In intestinal amoeba, cysts are characterized by having eight nuclei.

Control and test questions and assignments.

Draw a diagram of the life cycle of the amoeba and answer the questions below to test your knowledge.

1. Explain the systematics of amoeba enterica.

2. What is the size of the amoeba tissue?

3. What is the name of the main form of amoeba?

4. In which organ does the amoeba enterica parasitize?

Case 2. Structure and development cycle of trypanosomes.

Type. Sarcomastigophora - Sarcomastigophora

Junior type. Mastigophora - Mastigophora

Class. Zoosimonian predators – Zoomastigophorea

Category. Kinetoplastida - Kinetoplastida

Representative. The causative agent of African sleeping sickness -Trypanosoma gambiense

Required materials and equipment: Microscopy preparations prepared on trypanosomes, color and black-and-white slides, overhead projector, microscope, color tables depicting the structure and development cycle of trypanosomes.

Objective of the topic: To study the structure, development cycle and diseases caused by parasitic protozoa - trypanosomes.

Brief summary of the topic. Representatives of the genus Trypanosoma live in the blood, cerebrospinal fluid, and other organs of humans and vertebrates, secreting toxic substances into the blood and causing serious diseases. They are mostly colorless.

Trypanosomes are flat, rod-shaped or ribbon-like, 15-40 μm long. They have one flagellum located on the anterior side of the body, directed from the side to the back. The flagellum is attached to the ectoplasm by a thin, wavy membrane.

The basal body, or kinetoplast, is located in the endoplasm at the base of the spindle.

Trypanosomes infect humans and livestock, mainly in Africa, South and Central America, Asia, and Europe.

Among the trypanosomes, the causative agent of African sleeping sickness - Trypanosoma gambiense, the causative agent of Chagas disease - Trypanosoma cruzi, and the causative agent of Rhodesian sleeping sickness - Trypanosoma rhodesiense are well studied.

Trypanosoma gambiense is a parasite that causes a very serious disease called "sleeping sickness" that is widespread in Africa

In the first half of the 20th century, more than 1 million people died from this disease. The disease begins with an increase in body temperature, then gradually severe damage to the central nervous system is observed. The patient may fall asleep or, conversely, cannot sleep. If the disease is not treated in time, it can lead to death. The parasites enter the patients' blood, lymph nodes, and later, the cerebrospinal fluid.

The natural source of African sleeping sickness is antelopes, and the tsetse fly (Glossina palpalis) is the vector. The disease occurs only in areas where the tsetse fly is widespread. When the fly sucks the blood of a person, it infects the person with the parasite. In the fly's intestines, the parasites divide and reproduce asexually.

Trypanosoma cruzi - is the causative agent of Chagas disease, a dangerous disease in Latin America. Morphologically, it does not differ from the causative agent of African sleeping sickness. However, depending on the place of settlement, it has different forms. Trypanosoma, which parasitizes inside the cell, multiplies rapidly, forming pseudocysts. Parasites are virulent in the host and when cultivated artificially.

The carrier of Chagas disease is the blood-sucking tick Triatoma infestans. Trypanosomes live in the hindgut of the tick and develop over a period of 5-15 days. Once infected, the tick retains the trypanosomes throughout its life and is considered dangerous to humans. Usually, the parasites are transmitted to humans through various breaks and wounds in the skin and mucous membranes.

Triatoma mites attack humans, mainly at night, while they are sleeping, sucking blood from the mucous membranes of the lips, eyes, and nose. They often excrete feces contaminated with trypanosomes into the feeding area, and trypanosomes are easily transmitted to humans through broken skin. The parasites live in the cells of the skin and mucous membranes for 1-2 weeks, where they begin to multiply. Then, they leave the parasitic cells, enter the blood vessels, and spread throughout the body. During this period, the person's body temperature rises, and the parasites migrate to the cells of the heart, nervous system, digestive system, and reticuloendothelial organs, where they live.

Symptoms of the disease include fever, enlarged liver and spleen, and intestinal dysfunction. In children under 5 years of age, Chagas disease can be very severe and fatal.

According to some reports, up to 14% of patients die from this disease. The disease is also transmitted from mother to child through breast milk and blood transfusions. Chagas disease is most common in rural areas. In particular, in homes and in dirty places where sanitary and hygienic rules are not followed, the larvae of triatomine bugs develop freely.

Procedure for conducting work. For practical work, Trypanosoma equiperdum can be found. For work, dry preparations stained with Romanovsky-Giemsa can be used.

Take a drop of blood from a horse or mouse infected with trypanosomes, place it on a slide, and examine the slide through a small objective lens of a microscope. Note the small, round bodies. These are the erythrocytes in the horse or mouse's blood.

Trypanosomes look faint when examined with a small objective of a microscope. Look at this area of the preparation with a large objective. Here you will see red blood cells and long bodies between them. These bodies are trypanosomes.

When examining the structure of trypanosomes, one can see their nucleus, flagella, and the ciliated membrane at the edge of their body. This condition can also be observed in permanent preparations prepared from trypanosomes.

Control and test questions and assignments.

Draw the structure of a trypanosome in your sketchbook and answer the questions below.

1. Which animals are the natural source of African sleeping sickness?

2. What disease does Trypanosoma cruzi cause?

3. What is the shape and length of trypanosomes?

4. How many people died from which trypanosomiasis in the first half of the 20th century?

5. Trypanosomes live in the hindgut of which insect?

6. Which trypanosome is the carrier of the Triatoma canadensis?

7. List the species of parasitic kinetoplastids that infect humans and vertebrates.

8 How many species of trypanosomes have been well studied?

9. Name the parasite that lives in the hindgut of the snail and develops over a period of 5-15 days.

10. Where is the causative agent of Chagas disease spread and what percentage of people die from this disease?

11. What disease does trypanosomiasis, which is a parasite of cattle in South Asian countries, cause and what is its spreader?

12. Name the trypanosoma that infects camels, horses, and donkeys in Kazakhstan, Turkmenistan, and Uzbekistan and the disease it causes.

13. Describe the name of the trypanosoma that infects horses, its route of transmission, and the disease it causes.

Case 3. The structure and development cycle of Leishmania.

Type. Sarcomastigophora - Sarcomastigophora

Junior type. Mastigophora - Mastigophora

Class. Zoosimonian predators – Zoomastigophorea

Category. Kinetoplastida – Kinetoplastida

Representative. Cutaneous leishmaniasis – Leishmania tropisa

Required materials and equipment: Microscopy of Leishmania, microscope, color and black -and- white slides, overhead projector, tables showing the structure and development cycle

Objectives of the topic: To study the structure, development cycle, and diseases caused by Leishmania.

Summary of the topic. Members of the genus Leishmania are similar in structure to trypanosomiasis, but they parasitize on the skin and internal organs of humans and animals. When they parasitize inside a cell, they do not produce proteins and are inactive.

These parasites are extremely small (3-7 μm). They are round, oval cells with a single nucleus and kinetoplasts. Two types of leishmania are parasitic in humans. They are transmitted to humans in two ways: cutaneous leishmania - through the bite of a sandfly, and visceral leishmania - through the bite of a dog.

Tropical leishmania (Leishmania tropica) infects the skin of the face, hands, and feet of humans . Cutaneous leishmaniasis is widespread in Central Asia and the Caucasus. The parasite lives in skin cells and forms ulcers on the skin. The disease is divided into a chronic or acute form lasting a year or more (Ashgabat ulcer) and an acute form lasting 3-6 months (Penda ulcer).

Cutaneous leishmaniasis is also known as bad sore or pashshahor among the peoples of Central Asia.

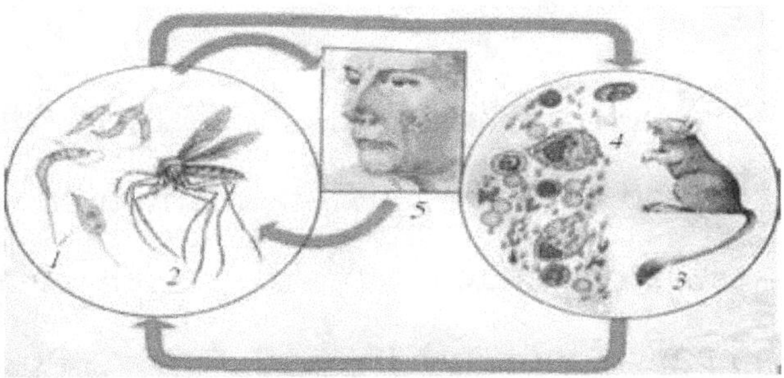

3. The development process of cutaneous leishmaniasis (*Leishmania tropica*):

1-leptomonad (filiform) form of Leishmania; 2-leishmania carrier iscabtopar; 3-rat (natural source); 4-leishmania without cilia in the blood cells of the affected skin; 5-human infected with leishmania.

Morphologically, leishmania occurs in two forms: intracellularly - without a flagella, and in the body of its carriers and when grown artificially - with a flagella. The flagellated phase of the life cycle of leishmania is called the leptomonad phase.

Visceral leishmaniasis is a severe disease characterized by frequent or intermittent fever. The causative agent of this leishmaniasis (Leishmania donovani) lives and multiplies as a parasite in the cytoplasm of endothelial cells in the human body - the liver, spleen, lymph nodes, and bone marrow (Figure 4).

When Leishmania multiplies, the number of parasites in one cell reaches 100-200 . After the cell is destroyed, they enter the blood with the lymph, enter new cells, and cause their destruction.

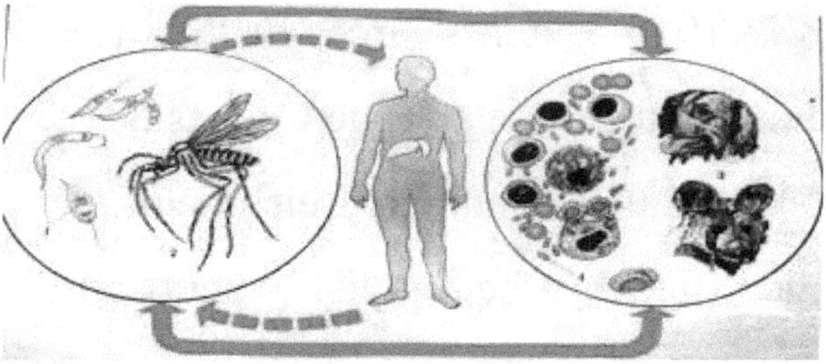

4 . The development process of the causative agent of internal leishmaniasis - Lieshmania donovani: *1-leptomonad (filiform) form of leishmania; 2-carrier of leishmania; 3-Natural sources of leishmania are dogs and other mammals; 4-In internal organs Leishmania without sebaceous glands.*

The causative agent of cutaneous leishmaniasis was first identified in Tashkent by the Russian physician PF Borovsky in 1882. A patient with internal leishmaniasis was first identified in the territory of the former Soviet

Union in 1909. Later, sources of the disease were found in Central Asia and the Caucasus.

Visceral leishmania (Leishmania donovani) was identified by the English scientist Leishman (military doctor W. Leeshman) in 1903 by isolating it from the spleen of a man who had died of this disease.

Leishmaniasis is a transmissible disease transmitted by sandflies of the genus Phlebotomus. When the sandflies suck the blood of an infected person, the leishmanias enter the insect's digestive tract and a long tentacle grows from the front end of the parasite, which means that the animal becomes a simple leptomaniac.

This insect, which is infected with the causative agent of leishmaniasis, transmits the parasites when it sucks the blood of a healthy person.

In general, leishmaniasis is widespread in several countries of North Africa, Southern Europe, and Southwest Asia. The disease is also widespread in the southern regions of Uzbekistan. The natural source of cutaneous leishmaniasis is rodents (sand rats and gerbils) and dogs, which are the reservoir hosts of leishmania.

These animals develop sores on their ears, noses, and other parts of their bodies where the tick can bite. The ticks hide in the burrows of rodents during the day, and at night they feed on the animals, infecting them with the disease.

There are two main forms of visceral leishmaniasis: Indian kala-azar and Mediterranean visceral leishmaniasis.

The skin color of the Indian Kala-Azari is dark, sometimes almost black. According to some scientists, this phenomenon is caused by a decrease in the activity of the adrenal glands, since leishmania is also found in the cortex of this gland.

Method of performing a smear test . For practical work, preparations prepared by smearing the skin of a dog with leishmaniasis or drying it from wounds on the skin can be used. Preparations can also be prepared from the wounds of a person with leishmania. The prepared preparations should be stained with Romanovsky-Giemza stain. Because Leishmania are very small, an immersion objective is used when examining the preparations.

Add a drop of cedar oil to the slide, place it on the microscope stage, then carefully lower the objective until it touches the cedar oil and focus. Parasites can be found both in the protoplasm of the spongy cells and outside the cells (if the cells were destroyed when the slide was prepared). Leishmania often grows in several cells, sometimes up to 100-200. When looking for Leishmania in a preparation, when stained with Ramanovsky-Giemsa stain, the protoplasm of the parasite is light blue or blue, and the nucleus is dark purple.

Examine the leishmania, find the nucleus, blepharoplasty and the root part of the hypha. If it is not possible to prepare the preparation, this can be done using ready-made permanent preparations. Draw a picture of Leishmania and answer the questions below.

Control and test questions and assignments.

1. How big are Leishmania?
2. How many species of Leishmania parasites infect humans?

3. Who was the first to identify cutaneous leishmaniasis?

4. Where and in which organs does visceral leishmania infect?

5. When Leishmania multiplies, how many parasites can be found in one cell?

6. Who identified visceral leishmaniasis?

7. Which insects transmit the leishmaniasis pathogen?

8. Which animals are the reservoir hosts of the causative agent of cutaneous leishmaniasis?

9. What do you understand by naturally occurring communicable diseases and who defined this concept?

11. Which family of parasites that transmit leishmaniasis belong to?

12. What are the forms of cutaneous and visceral leishmaniasis?

13. In which areas can the Kala-azar trigger be encountered?

2-PRACTICAL TRAINING

Topic: The structure and development of parasitic unicellular organisms - Giardia, Trichomonas, and Eimeria.

Case 1. The structure and reproduction cycle of Giardia .

Type. Sarcomastigophora - Sarcomastigophora

Junior type. Mastigophora - Mastigophora

Class. Zoosimonian predators – Zoomastigophorea

Category. Diploma - Diplomonad

And a kil. Giardia - Lamblia intestinalis

Required materials and equipment: Microscopy of Leishmania, microscope, color and black -and- white slides, overhead projector, tables showing the structure and development..

The purpose of the lesson . To study the structure of Giardia , the cycle of growth and development .

Short content . Diploma category A guide to the delicate digestive system of dogs The species belonging to the genus Lyamblia are the main species . About 40 types of Giardia are unique . One of the most common types is Lamblia intestinalis . Lamblia, Russian death DF Lamblia sh a r a fig a put .

Giardia occurs in the form of cysts in the wild cichlid . Vegetative shoots are oval , 12-15 μm long , 8-10 μm wide (5 - th cm) .

On the front of the body of Giardia there is a disk, which serves to attach to the intestinal epithelium. In the middle of the body there are two supporting threads - axostyles. With the help of axostyles, the body of the parasite is divided into two symmetrical segments, each of which has a single nucleus. In the front part of the axostyles there are several blepharoplasts, which provide energy to 3 pairs of flagella. The fourth pair of flagella lies behind the axostyles.

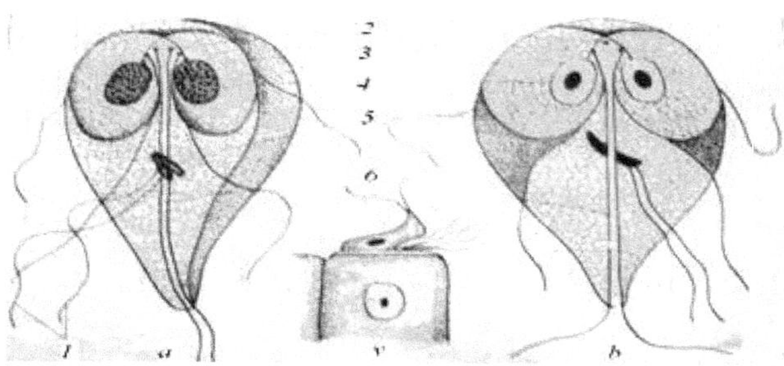

5. Structure of intestinal giardia (Lamblia intestinalis) : *a) lateral view, b) ventral view, c) giardia attached to epithelial tissue: 1-cluster; 2-basal body; 3-sac; 4-nucleus; 5-parabasal body; 6-axostyle.*

The parasite does not have digestive organs. Therefore, it feeds osmotically. The method of reproduction is asexual, it occurs by longitudinal division. The cysts of Giardia are oval in shape, reaching a length of 10-14 μm. A two-layered shell is clearly visible. Immature cysts have 2 nuclei, and mature ones have 4 nuclei.

The life cycle of Giardia is simple, with the life cycle consisting of alternating vegetative and cystic forms of the parasite. The vegetative form lives and multiplies in the duodenum of humans. In experimentally infected animals, Giardia have been found in the upper parts of the small intestine. Some of them, encased in cysts, are released into the environment and are considered a source of infection of humans with giardiasis. The source of infection of giardiasis pathogens is a sick person and parasite carriers.

Giardiasis is widespread, with parasites found in about 10% of the population. Young children are most commonly affected by Giardiasis.

In the 1920s, giardiasis was widespread in almost all countries of the world. According to most doctors and scientists, giardia is considered a conditionally pathogenic organism. Because parasites are found in healthy people, and when their number increases in the intestine, they change the intestinal function. For this reason, the absorption of substances slows down. People develop recurrent, that is, recurring, cases of enteritis, enterocolitis, and sometimes cholecystitis.

Prof N.A. Dekhkonhojaeva examined the small intestine of naturally and experimentally infected animals and found parasites in the mucous membrane and submucosal layer, as well as in the intestinal villi. In this case, the mucous membrane of the intestinal wall was inflamed, but no ulcers were formed. According to the doctor, the degree of changes in the intestinal mucosa depends on the duration of the disease.

The symptoms of the disease are similar to those of other intestinal diseases. Therefore, the main indicator of the diagnosis of giardiasis should be the detection of parasites. Vegetative forms of the parasite are found in the duodenal fluid. The presence of parasite cysts is determined by staining the patient's stool with iodine. Giardia cysts are released into the environment with their feces and can survive for weeks. A healthy person is infected with parasitic cysts through food, drinking water, or dirty hands. After entering the digestive tract, the cysts turn into a vegetative form in the duodenum.

To prevent disease, it is necessary to follow preventive rules. To do this, wash fruits and vegetables thoroughly, boil water before drinking, store cooked food and drinking water in closed containers, fight mosquitoes and flies, wash hands before eating and after using the toilet, timely check up on parasite carriers, especially those working in food factories and kindergartens, treat sick people, and disinfect toilets. necessary.

Procedure. Examine the Giardia preparation with an immersion microscope. Pay attention to the shape of the body and the symmetrical arrangement of organelles in pairs, find the axostyle, nucleus, adherent disk, and flagella.

Control and test questions and assignments.

Draw a picture of Giardia and answer the questions below.

1. In which organs does Giardia parasitize and multiply?

2. What percentage of the population is infected with giardiasis?

3. What is the genus of Giardia and how many species are there?

4. What are the stages in the life cycle of Giardia?

5. What is the function of the disc on the front of the Giardia body?

6. How is Giardia transmitted to humans?

7. Who discovered Giardia in Uzbekistan?

Task 2. Study the structure, development cycle, and diseases caused by Trichomonas.

Type. Sarcomastigophora - Sarcomastigophora

Junior type. Mastigophora - Mastigophora

Class. Animal-like predators – Zomastigophorea

Category: Trichomonads – Trichomonadida

Representative. Intestinal trichomonas - Trichomonas hominis

Required materials and equipment: Microscopy of Trichomonas, immersion microscope, cedar oil and black-and-white slides, overhead projector, color tables showing the structure and development cycle.

Objective of the topic: To study the structure, development cycle, and harm caused to humans by Trichomonas.

Summary of the topic. Trichomonas are the causative agents of trichomonadosis, and 3 types of them parasitize humans: Intestinal Trichomonas - Trichomonas hominis, Vaginal Trichomonas - Trichomonas vaginalis, and Oral Trichomonas - Trichomonas tenax.

Intestinal Trichomonas parasitizes in the large intestine of humans. Vaginal, that is, urogenital Trichomonas parasitizes in the urinary and genital tracts of women and men. The body of Trichomonas is oval in shape, narrowed in the posterior part. Its length is from 5-10 μm to 15-30 μm. In the anterior part, a spherical nucleus is located, and in front of the nucleus lies a blepharoplast.

Like other representatives of the class of zoosimonous protozoa, protozoa also perform the function of organelles of movement. The number of protozoa is 4-5, one of which is directed backward along the protozoan membrane. There are digestive vacuoles in the cytoplasm. The body of Trichomonas has a long, basal core, the axostyle, and a wavy membrane along its edge (Fig. 6). The ciliated membrane of vaginal Trichomonas and oral Trichomonas is short. Trichomonas feed in two ways, that is, they absorb nutrients from the entire surface of the body - osmotically or through the cellular mouth - cytostome, that is, by the method of capture. However, the cystostomy of vaginal Trichomonas has not been identified so far. Trichomonas reproduce asexually by longitudinal division - mitosis. It is not known whether cysts form.

Intestinal Trichomonas does not cause serious diseases in humans, but it can accelerate the development of colitis. Intestinal Trichomonas is transmitted through contaminated food or water. To diagnose intestinal Trichomonas, the patient's stool is examined under a microscope to identify vegetative forms.

Urogenital (vaginal) trichomonas is widespread. They parasitize the urinary tract of men and women. The incidence of the disease is 20–40% in women and 15% in men. Urogenital (vaginal) trichomonas is transmitted as a result of poor personal hygiene and during sexual intercourse. Vaginal trichomonas causes severe and difficult-to-treat diseases in humans. To make a diagnosis, a swab is taken from the patient's urinary and genital tract and examined under a microscope.

The pathogenicity of oral Trichomonas has not been determined. However, it is more common in people with oral and dental diseases. Therefore, special attention should be paid to methods for detecting oral Trichomonas in dental clinics.

It is necessary to take preventive measures such as washing hands thoroughly before eating , storing water used for cooking in a closed container , and observing good hygiene rules during the meal .

Methodology of work . Immersion microscope with objective lens Take a look at the preparation of trichomonates painted in Arnold 's method . You can see that the nucleus of the parasite is in the same shape as before . Next to him , there was a long crack in the room .

The side of the body It 's a clear wave of the wave that you know .. It looks blue and white . After completing the preparation , visualize the room in which you are sleeping .

Trichomonas vaginalis: 1- ciliated membrane; 2- anterior cilia; 3- blepharoplast; 4- nucleus; 5- basal axostyle.

Control and test questions and assignments.

Draw the shape of the triangle in a notebook and write it down .

1. What is the length of the triangle with the length of the triangle ?

3. Where is the nucleus of Trichomonas located ?

4. What are the characteristics of Trichomonas ?

5. What is the meaning of trichomoniasis ?

6. Does Tricho mone eat a lot ?

7. What types of trichomonads are different in humans ?

7. Does internal trichomoniasis cause pain ?

3. STRUCTURE OF THE EYM ERA DEVELOPMENT CYCLE

Type. Apikomplexlar - Apicomplexa
Category. Coccidial a r - Coccidia
Subcategory. Eimeriina - Eimeriina
Representative: Eimeria magna - Eimeria magna

Required materials and equipment: Coccidiag a te micro - parameters , gy, their structure and life cycle are displayed on a nr a ng wall , di o pr oe ctor , micro sco pe , hand loup Tweezers , binoculars , clamps , objects and toys , wire probes , wire mesh , cuvette , saline solution , chicken , rabbit test , wet preparation .

The purpose of the lesson . To study the structure , development cycle and the health of the erythrocyte in the intestinal epithelial cells of the rabbit .

Summary of the topic. The class of sporozoans includes more than 4,000 species, all of which are parasitic in various internal organs of invertebrates and vertebrates, including humans. Therefore, their development has become complex, and new features have emerged, such as the ability to live in a variety of environmental conditions, change hosts, and reproduce asexually and sexually. Their motile organelles, contractile and digestive vacuoles are not developed, and they form spores by being wrapped in a protective shell.

The class of sporozoans is divided into the families Coccidia and Gregarinidae. Members of the coccidia family are parasites of animals and humans, causing dangerous diseases.

The phylum Coccidia is in turn divided into several subphyla.

Members of the suborder Eimeria (Eimeriina) are parasitic mainly in the intestinal epithelial cells of vertebrate organs, namely the intestines and liver. Almost each species of coccidia is parasitic only in a specific species of animal. Adult coccidia are non-motile.

Young sporozoites and merozoites, which are elongated in shape, are actively moving. The reproduction of coccidia is characterized by the correct division of sexual and asexual stages. Species of the genus Eimeria mainly parasitize cattle, sheep, goats, rabbits and poultry. The development of coccidia is complex, and in all animals there is one type, and it goes through three stages of development (schizogony, gametogeny and sporogony). The life cycle of Eimeria magna, a parasite that lives in the intestinal epithelial cells of rabbits, namely the intestines and liver, is described below (Figure 7).

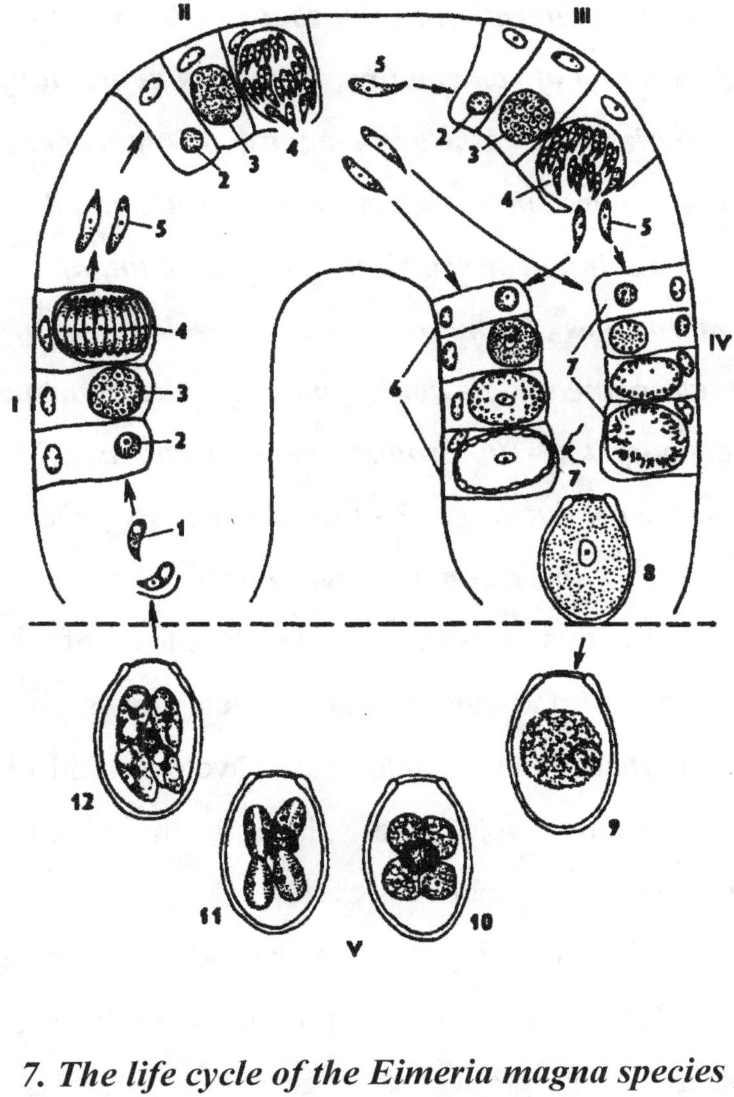

7. The life cycle of the Eimeria magna species , which belongs to the Eimeria family :

I - first generation of schizogony , II - second generation of schizogony , III - third generation of schizogony , IV - gametogony , V - sporogony : 1 - sporozoites , 2 - uninuclear schizont , 3 - multinuclear schizont , 4 - production of merozoites , 5 - merozoites , 6 - development of macrogametes , 7 - development of microgametes , 8 - oocyst , 9-10 - production of sporoblasts ,11 - spore production , 12 - four spore cysts (each spore contains two spores) .

In this way , the development of the schizogony and gagametogony cycles takes place in internal organs (endogenous cycle) , and the sporogenous cycle takes place in the external environment (exogenous cycle) .

Shiz ogynia , , the period of asexual reproduction , and sexual reproduction of the same organ . The product is ingested by animals , including rabbits , along with food or water . Oo cyst contains 4 spores and 2 spores per cyst . Rabbit drink a The outer layer of the oocyst has melted , the skin of the spore has cracked and the spore has come out .

The spores penetrate the epithelial cells in the arterioles and , having grown , increase in size , and the nucleus divides into several (8-60) segments . The nuclei divide into several cytoplasmic segments and form new offspring , i.e. merospores .

When the virus leaves the intestinal epithelial cells , it enters the male epithelial cells and produces the second generation asexually . In this way , after 4-5 months of asexual reproduction , sexual cells (gametes) are produced in the human body .

During gametogenesis (sexual reproduction) , a group of germ cells (asexual) enter the epithelial cell and form a group of micro gamete cells . Each microgamete has one microgamete , and each microgamete is small , elongated , with a pair of cells .It will be fine .

More than 10 types of coccidials are found in cattle , about 10 types in sheep and goats , 10 types in rabbits , and 8 types in sheep . Eimiria sardinae and Isospora species are the most common species of the occidental species .

Coccidiosis is a disease caused by coccidia . This disease is especially dangerous for young rabbits , causing them to die in droves .

Procedure . Rabbit or chicken feces infected with coccidia are taken and placed in a glass or a container with a saturated physiological solution . After a certain time , the oocysts of the Neisseria meningitidis are placed in a container with a looped wire and placed on the solution as a specimen .

The magnification of a microscope With the help of the objective , you can find microwaves and microwaves by moving the device . Draw a picture of different rivers in a book .

Control and test questions and assignments.

According to the microscope , mononuclear schiz o ont , multinuclear schiz o ont , merozo itl a r , micro o g a m o n t , m a c r o g a m e t a l a rv a Carefully inspect the system and draw the correct name of the riv o jl a nish cycle of the eim e riya in a book and write it down .

1. Who is the coccidial group and what is the cause of the disease ?

2. According to Eym e riyal a r riv o jl a nishig a nd a yd a vrl a Is that it ?

3. What is the difference between science and technology ?

4. What is the purpose of the sport ?

5. What is the meaning of the riyal ?

6. How many types of money do sheep and goats have ?

7. Eimeria Describe the systematics of the magna species .

8. Is it possible to express the quality of the products in real terms ?

3-PRACTICAL TRAINING

Subject: Parasite one from cells - the structure and development processes of the malaria parasite, ichthyophthirius, and balantidium

1 - CASE. STRUCTURE AND DEVELOPMENT CYCLE OF THE MALARIA PARASITE

SYSTEMATIC STATUS OF THE MALARIA PARASITE

Type. Apicomplexes - Apicomplexa

Class. Sporozoea - Sporozoea

Category. Coccidia - Coccidiida

Subfamily. Bloodspores - Haemosporina

Representative. The malaria parasite is Plasmodium vivax

Required materials and equipment. Microscopy prepared from the blood of a person infected with the malaria parasite, a microscope with an immersion objective. Tables showing the structure and development cycle of the malaria parasite.

Objectives of the topic: To gain an understanding of malaria parasites, to study the structure, development cycle, and disease caused by the three-day malaria parasite (Plasmodium vivax).

Brief summary of the topic . Representatives of the subfamily of blood sporozoites parasitize the red blood cells of humans and warm-blooded animals. This subfamily includes about 100 species.

Blood sporozoites are intracellular parasites similar to coccidia, but their life cycle occurs in several hosts. The most important representative of this subfamily, the malaria plasmodium, which causes malaria in humans, develops in two hosts. While asexual reproduction and macro- and microgametocyte stages occur in human red blood cells, sexual development occurs in the malaria mosquito (Anopheles). The spores that spread malaria among humans are called plasmodium.

This disease was known even before our era. Malaria plasmodiums were first discovered in 1879 by the Russian scientist V.I. Afanasyev and in 1880 by the French scientist Alphonse Laverne. The fact that malaria is spread by mosquitoes was determined in 1895 by the English scientist R. Ross and the Italian scientist J. Grassi.

There are 4 main types of malaria parasites that infect humans:

1. Plasmodium vivax is a three-day malaria pathogen, meaning the fever recurs every 48 hours.

2. Plasmodium malariae is a four-day malaria pathogen, meaning the fever recurs every 72 hours.

3. Plasmodium falciparum is a tropical malaria pathogen that attacks every 24-48 hours and is often very severe.

4. Plasmodium ovale is a three-day malaria pathogen, meaning the fever recurs every 48 hours. This malaria pathogen is very rarely found in tropical Africa and Asian countries.

The first three species are widespread in tropical and subtropical countries. The development of the three-day malaria plasmodium - Plasmodium vivax - is carried out in a funnel (Figure 7).

When a mosquito infected with the parasite bites a person, the sporozoites in the mosquito's saliva are transferred into the blood. These sporozoites travel through the blood to the liver and spleen. Here they begin to feed and multiply, that is, their nuclei divide into several, then the cytoplasm divides into several, depending on the size of the nucleus, and the next generation of the parasite, merozoites, is formed. Later, these merozoites enter red blood cells and feed on hemoglobin plasma.

This happens 48 hours after the merozoite enters the erythrocyte and at the same time the person gets malaria. The reason is that along with thousands of merozoites, a toxic substance called melanin is released into the blood plasma and poisons the blood. The merozoites in the blood plasma then enter healthy erythrocytes and begin asexual development anew. In some cases, sexual individuals - gametocytes - are formed in the blood of a patient whose reproduction is restored by schizogony, that is, female macrogametocytes and male microgametocytes are formed from merozoites inside erythrocytes.

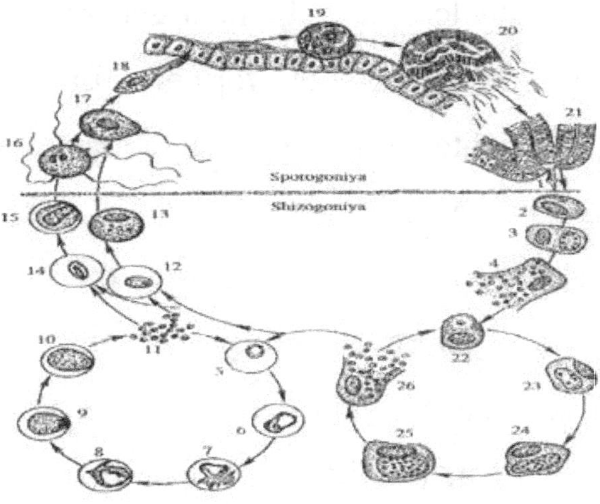

***8. Scheme of the development cycle of the malaria parasite** : 1-merozoites released from the salivary gland of the malaria mosquito into human blood; 2,3-multiplication of sporozoites in liver cells; 4-formation of merozoites from sporozoites by schizogony; 5-11-multiplication of merozoites in erythrocytes by schizogony; 12,13-macrogametocyte maturation; 14,15-microgametocyte maturation; 16,17-formation of macrogametes and microgametes and their fusion; 18-entry of zygotes - ookinetes into the*

cells of the mosquito's gut; 19, 20-formation of sporozoites and their release into the mosquito's body cavity; 21-transmission of sporozoites into the mosquito's salivary gland; 22-26-development of the mosquito in human cells.

The subsequent development of gametocytes occurs in the midgut of the Anopheles mosquito. When the Anopheles mosquito sucks the blood of a person infected with malaria, the gametocytes are transferred to the mosquito. As a result of the development of microgametocytes inside the mosquito, 5-6 microgametes with 4-8 zygotes are formed. The nuclei of the macrogametocytes also multiply and become macrogametes. These macrogametes and microgametes fuse to form a zygote. The zygote is motile and is called an ookinete.

The ookinete penetrates the wall of the mosquito's stomach, wraps itself in an elastic membrane, and becomes an oocyst. As the oocyst grows, its nucleus divides several times, each nuclear division being surrounded by cytoplasm, resulting in thousands of tiny, zygote-like sporozoites.

Then the oocyst membrane ruptures, and the number of sporozoites inside reaches 10,000. They fall into the body cavity of the mosquito, and through the hemolymph fluid they reach all organs, including the mosquito's salivary glands, where they multiply. When such infected mosquitoes bite a healthy person, the sporozoites, along with the mosquito's saliva, enter the human bloodstream.

Sporozoites are uninucleate, elongated filaments, 10-15 μm long. There are more than 150 species of mosquitoes of the genus Anopheles on Earth, of which 50 species are of epidemiological importance. In addition to being the main host of the malaria parasite, the mosquito is also considered the vector of malaria.

Malaria is widespread in tropical and subtropical regions of the world, killing thousands of people each year. Malaria was eradicated in our republic in the 1960s.

Procedure. A smear from the blood of a person with three days of malaria is smeared onto a slide and observed under the immersion objective of a microscope. Here, white and red blood cells can be seen. Erythrocytes infected with Plasmodium vivax are smaller than those of uninfected individuals.

If cedar oil is added to the preparation, the nucleus of the malaria parasite will turn cherry-colored, and its protoplasm will turn sky-blue.

Find the first developmental stage of the schizont and the vacuole inside it from the preparation being observed. Observe the stage when the schizont is preparing for division. There is no vacuole during this stage. Its body is oval in shape and has no pseudopodia. It reproduces by division through schizogony. During this stage, there are 12-18 merozoites, their protoplasm is light blue and the nucleus is cherry-colored.

Control and test questions and assignments .

1. Who are the representatives of the suborder Consporales parasitic on?

2. How many species are included in the suborder Consporales?

3. Who and when were malaria parasites first discovered?

4. Who discovered that mosquitoes spread malaria?

5. How many types of malaria parasites infect humans?

3 – WORK. STRUCTURE AND DEVELOPMENT CYCLE OF BALANTHIUM

SYSTEMATIC STATUS OF BALANTIDIUM

Type. Infusoria - Ciliophora

Class: Ciliates - Ciliata

Junior class. Infusoria with cilia - Holotricha

Category. Trichostomatida - Trichostomatida

Representative. Balantidia - Balantidium coli

Required materials and equipment: Prepared micropreparations for Balantidia and Ichthyophthirius, color tables showing the structure and development cycle of Balantidia and Ichthyophthirius, microscope.

Objectives of the topic. To provide an understanding of the harmful effects of Balantidia in the intestines of humans and pigs, and the parasitic nature of Ichthyophthirius in fish . To study the structure, development cycle, and harm of Balantidia and Ichthyophthirius.

Summary of the topic. Many species of the ciliate subclass, which belong to the class of ciliates, are parasitic in various organs of various invertebrates and vertebrates. Of the parasitic ciliate infusoria, the harmfulness of Balantidium coli, which belongs to the subclass of ciliates, is especially great. Balantidium coli is mainly parasitic in the large intestine of humans (Figure 8).

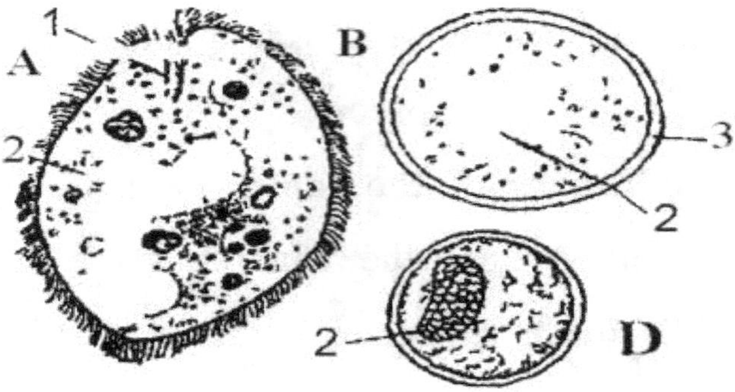

9. Balantidium coli infusoria: A-active swimming form; B-unstained cyst; D-stained cyst; 1-mouth opening; 2-macronucleus; 3-cyst shell.

This species or a similar species also infects the large intestine of pigs, hogs, and rats. Balantidia causes lesions in the intestine and causes balantidiasis, a dangerous disease similar to bloody diarrhea.

The shape of the balantidia is oval, bean-shaped, round, and ovoid, with the anterior side slightly narrowed and the posterior side slightly widened. The body of the infusoria is covered with a pellicle, under which lies a layer of clear ectoplasm. There are 2 nuclei located in the rough endoplasm, the large bean-shaped nucleus is called the macronucleus, and the nucleolus located to the right is called the micronucleus. The body is covered on the surface with small, one-meter-long cilia. The cilia perform the function of movement and capture food. The mouth on the front side - the cystostome - is connected to a short throat - the cytopharynx.

The length of the balantidia ranges from 40 to 150 μm and the width from 20 to 70 μm. The balantidia have 2 vacuoles, one located on the anterior side of the body and the other on the posterior side.

Balantidia also have the ability to form cysts. In this case, balantidia lower their cilia and form a dense two-layered cyst. The cysts are large, reaching a diameter of 50-60 μm. Balantidia divide into two and reproduce asexually and sexually.

Because balantidium is also a parasite in the intestines of pigs, mice, and rats. The cysts of the parasite are excreted in the feces of pigs, and people ingest these cysts and become ill with balantidium.

The disease is caused by the ingestion of Balantidium cysts by unwashed hands, which are the result of poor hygiene. The parasite is released from the cysts in the rectum. Balantidium is most often contracted by workers on pig farms and sausage factories.

Balantidiasis mainly affects weaned pigs. The disease can be acute or chronic. In the acute form, the affected animal has a high temperature and diarrhea mixed with blood and mucus. In the chronic form, there is a lack of appetite and periodic recurrence of diarrhea. Most pigs infected with balantidiasis die.

4-PRACTICAL TRAINING

Topic: Parasitic flatworms - the structure and development of liver flukes, lancelet flukes, and blood flukes.

Case 1. The structure and development cycle of the liver fluke.

Type. Flatworms - Plathelminthes

Class. Suckers – Trematoda

Category. Fasciolidae - Fasciolida

Subfamily. Fasciolata - Fasciolata

Representative. Common liver fluke - Fasciola hepatica

Materials and equipment needed for the exercise. Prepared preparations on the structure of the liver fluke's digestive, excretory, and reproductive organs, live liver flukes, fixed liver flukes, hand loupes, binoculars, microscopes, forceps, slides, specimens and coverslips, Petri dishes, color tables depicting the structure and development cycle of the liver fluke.

Objective of the topic. The common liver fluke , which is a parasite in the liver and bile ducts of humans and livestock, **Studying** its unique structure and adaptations to parasitism, its development cycle, and the disease it causes.

Summary of the topic. Currently, the class of trematodes, that is, flukes, includes more than 5,000 species. Almost all of them are parasitic in various tissues and organs of humans and farmed animals.

The development of trematodes, however, is more complex, and their development occurs through the development of hosts and joints. Thus, flukes develop through one, sometimes two intermediate hosts. In such cases, their first intermediate hosts are, of course, mollusks living in water and on land. The second intermediate (additional) hosts can be various insects (ants), their larvae (dragonfly larvae), fish, and representatives of aquatic and terrestrial organisms.

The main hosts of tapeworms are various mammals, birds, and other vertebrates, as well as humans.

In our republic, two main types of liver flukes are parasitic in farm animals and humans: the common liver fluke (Fasciola hepatica) and the giant liver fluke (Fasciola gigantica). The common liver fluke (Fasciola hepatica) usually infects small and large cattle, and sometimes the liver and bile ducts of other animals and humans. The length of the liver fluke is 2-3.6 cm, and the width is up to 5 12 mmcm. (Figure 9).

The liver fluke is considered a biohelminth, meaning that two hosts are involved in its development. In this case, an intermediate host is required to pass the initial stage of development, and a definitive host is required for the parasite to fully develop.

The freshwater snail (Lymnaea truncatula), a small gastropod mollusk that lives in freshwater, is the intermediate host of the liver fluke, while sheep, goats, cattle, horses, camels, pigs, rodents, and sometimes humans are the primary hosts of the parasite.

Currently, 18 species of freshwater mollusks have been identified as intermediate hosts for fasciolala.

The liver fluke is a parasite, and one liver fluke can lay up to a million eggs in a week. Under favorable conditions in the external environment, after 17-18 days, a motile larva, covered with tiny cilia, emerges. The miracidia swim freely in the water for 2-3 days and, having found an intermediate host - a gastropod mollusk - for further development, pierces the mollusk shell with its proboscis and enters it. These larvae then settle in the mollusk's liver, shed their ciliated outer layer, and develop into the next larval stage, the sporocyst, which takes on a shell-like shape.

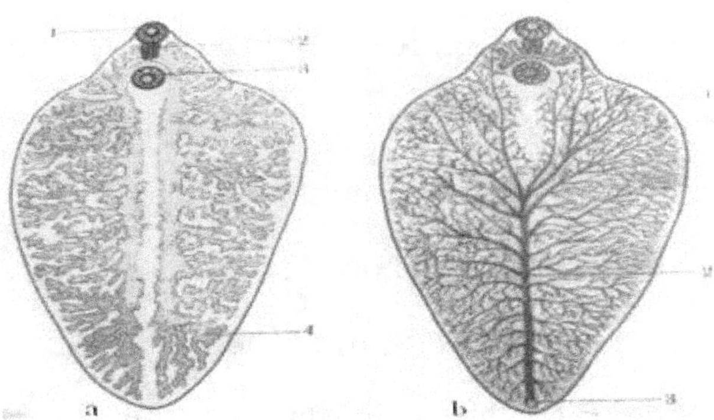

10. Digestive and excretory organs of Fasciola hepatica: *a) digestive organs: 1-oral sucker and mouth; 2-larynx; 3-abdominal sucker; 4-branched intestine;*

b) excretory organs: 1-protonephridia; 2-central excretory duct; 3-excretory pore.

The embryonic cells inside the sporocyst multiply by parthenogenesis (without fertilization) and produce the next generation of larvae, the radii. The radii have a small pouch-like intestine. 10-15 radii develop in one sporocyst. The sporocyst ruptures and the radii emerge into the body of the mollusk. Radiata are more complex in structure, with a mouth, an unbranched rectum, and egg (embryonic) cells inside.

Such radiolarians break through the sporocyst shell and continue their development as independent larvae. Radiolarians live inside the mollusk for 2-2.5 months. Elongated radiolarians also reproduce parthenogenetically, producing cercariae, the next larval stage of the liver fluke. Cercariae differ sharply from radiolarians in that they have an egg-shaped body, two suckers, namely the oral and abdominal suckers, a midgut divided into two branches, a well-developed excretory system, a rudimentary genital tract, and a muscular tail with a larval organ at the posterior end.

Cercariae swim in the water with this tail. So, cercariae are somewhat similar to adult liver flukes. Cercariae exit the mollusk's body into the water through a hole in the body of the radion. Cercariae do not feed like myracids. It swims in the water for a certain time (24-48 hours), then curls up, loses its tail, and turns into a shell, a cyst, which it sheds, and then into a later larval stage called the juvenile stage.

Adolescents float on the surface of the water or, often clinging to aquatic plants, remain alive for long periods of time by sinking to the bottom.

Adolescents are considered to be infectious. They are transmitted to the final host organism through feces and water. In the intestine, the cyst shell dissolves, the young parasite attaches to the intestinal walls of the animal and travels through the blood capillaries to the liver and bile ducts, where it matures and the above life cycle is repeated (Fig. 11).

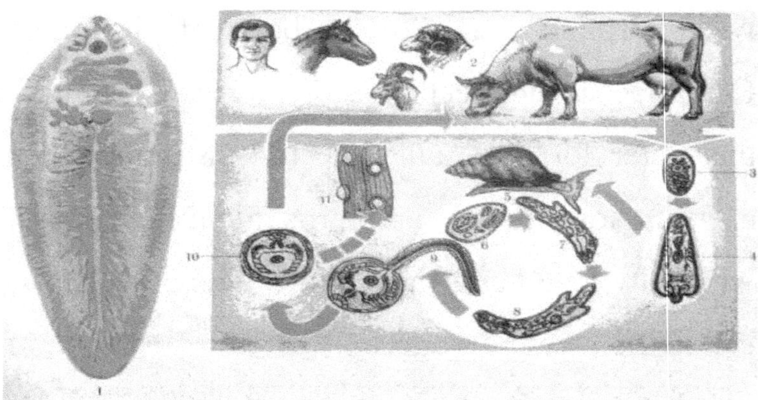

11. Schematic of the life cycle of Fasciola hepatica: *1-sexual adult form (mary); 2-final hosts; 3-egg; 4-miracidia; 5-intermediate host-mollusk; 6-sporocyst; 7-young redia; 8-mature*

redia; 9-cercaria; 10-adolescentia; 11-adolescentia attached to the grass .

Thus, it takes 60-90 days for a miracidium to enter the mollusk's body and develop into a cercariae. Reproducing parthenogenetically, one miracidium can produce up to 600-800 cercariae. The juveniles that enter the body of the primary host reach sexual maturity after 2.5-4 months and live in the body of the primary host from an average of 10-12 months to 3-5 years, sometimes more than 10 years. The liver fluke feeds mainly on blood and liver tissue, causing great harm to its host. This parasite causes severe liver disease due to the accumulation of lime in the bile ducts of the liver and their blockage.

The disease caused by the liver fluke is called fascioliasis. The causative agents of this disease are widespread in swamps and meadows with abundant fresh water. In particular, fascioliasis is widespread when sick animals are kept in one place for a long time without changing pastures. This is because a sick animal continuously releases parasite eggs in its feces. In general, fascioliasis is widespread on Earth.

Humans can also get fascioliasis. People can become infected by accidentally drinking water from ponds, lakes, and streams that contain invisible liver fluke larvae, or by eating unwashed seaweed.

In general, to avoid getting sick with this disease, people should first of all avoid drinking running water without boiling it, and thoroughly wash and eat herbs growing in water and marshes. Sick people should, of course, be treated with the drug chloroxylenol. Thus, it takes 60-90 days for the miracidium to enter the mollusk's body and turn into cercariae. Reproduction is parthenogenetic, and up to 600-800 cercariae are produced from one brood. The juveniles, having entered the body of the main host, reach sexual maturity after 2.5-4 months and live in the body of the main host from an average of 10-12 months to 3-5 years, sometimes more than 10 years. Liver fluke feeds mainly on blood and liver tissue, causing severe damage to its host. This parasite causes severe liver disease by causing the bile ducts in the liver to become blocked and calcified.

An animal infected with liver fluke loses its appetite, becomes lethargic, and produces less milk. The affected animal's abdomen, chest, and throat atrophy, and tumors develop. To treat cattle infected with fascioliasis, they are given drugs (anthelmintics) that kill fasciolae and expel them from the animal's body.

Procedure. Examine the liver of a cow or sheep that has been infested with liver flukes.

Note the location of the liver fluke in the liver. Place the alcohol-fixed or live liver flukes in a Petri dish using forceps or a microscope slide and examine them under a magnifying glass, noting their size, color, and the bilateral symmetry of their body from the dorsal to the ventral sides, and whether they are flattened. Examine the mouth and abdominal suckers. Measure the length of its body.

To study the internal organs, specially stained micropreparations are used, showing the digestive, excretory, and reproductive organs.

In the digestive system of a liverworm, note the mouth opening located between the mouthparts at the front of the body, the pharynx, and the two main and numerous small branches of the intestine that begin after it. To see the digestive system more clearly, the food in the intestines is removed and sent away. To do this, the liverworm is pressed from the back with a finger, facing the front, or it is placed in cold water. Then, a solution of Prussian blue is taken with a syringe or pipette and injected through the mouth.

When examining stained slides of the efferent organ under a microscope, note the presence of the main efferent tube and the small collecting tubes around it.

When observing the reproductive organs, first find the paired testes located in the middle of the body, and the sperm ducts leading from them to the cirrus. Note that the cirrus lies inside the cirrus sac. Observe the yolk sacs on both sides of the body, and the longitudinal and transverse tubes that join them to the body of the Melis.

Examine stained slides of liver fluke larvae - myracidium, radii, cercariae, and adolescariae -

through small and large objectives of a microscope and study their structure.

To observe live myracidium, liver fluke eggs are placed in a Petri dish filled with tap water and kept in a thermostat at +28-30 ^{0} C for 14-15 days. The top of the Petri dish containing the eggs should be covered with black paper.

Before the start of the exercise, the container with the liver fluke eggs is placed in a bright place for several hours. The larvae will soon hatch from such eggs. If you take a few drops of water from a Petri dish, put them on the glass slide, cover it with a coverslip, and look through the small objective of the microscope, you can see the moving liver fluke larvae - the larvae.

Control and test questions and assignments .

Draw pictures in your album depicting the digestive, reproductive systems, and developmental cycle of a liver fluke and answer the questions below.

1. Provide information about the definitive and intermediate hosts of the liver fluke.

2. How many types of liver flukes are parasitic in livestock in Uzbekistan?

3. What are the larval stages in the development of a liver fluke?

4. How many eggs does a liver fluke lay in a week?

5. How many days does it take for a liver fluke egg to hatch into a larva in the external environment?

6. How many radicles mature in one sporocyst?

7. How long do radiolarians live inside a mollusk?

8. How long does it take for a liver fluke larva - a miracidium - to transform into a cercariae after entering a mollusk?

9. How many cercariae are produced from a single liver fluke embryo as a result of parthenogenetic reproduction?

10. How long does it take for a juvenile liver fluke to reach adulthood after entering its primary host?

11. How long does an adult liver fluke live on average in its primary host?

12. Explain the development of a liver fluke, starting from the egg.

13. What disease does the liver fluke cause?

Case 2. The structure and development cycle of the two-sucking lancelet.

Type. Other worms - Plathelminthes

Class: Flukes – Trematoda

Category. Plagiorchiidae - Plagiorchiida

Family: Disrocoeliidae

Representative. Lancetsimon's two-sucking - Disrocoelium dendritisum

Required materials and equipment . Color tables depicting the structure and development cycle of the lancelet, prepared stained preparations of the lancelet, live and alcohol-fixed lancelet from sheep or cattle liver, magnifying glass with tripod, microscope, forceps, specimen and coverslips, preparation slides.

Objective: To study the structure and development cycle of the Lancetsimon bivalves.

Summary of the topic. The lancelet tapeworm or dendritic tapeworm (Dicrocoelium dendriticum), a member of the class Dicrocoelidae, is a liver fluke that infects cattle and other vertebrates, and sometimes humans. It is also called the lancelet tapeworm because its body resembles a surgical blade (lancet).

The body of the two-sucking lancelet is elongated, about 5 15 mmcm long. The suckers are located close to each other. Although they are similar in structure to the liverworm, there are some differences. In particular, their intestines, which are located along the edge of the body, are not curved and end in a visible part at the end of the body. Two round testicles are located behind the abdominal sucker, followed by a single round egg.

The life cycle of the lancelet tapeworm involves three hosts (Figure 12). The primary host is a variety of vertebrates and sometimes humans, the first intermediate host is a terrestrial mollusk (Nelicella Zebrina and others), and the secondary host is ants (Formica, Proformica).

When mollusks feed, they also swallow the eggs of two protozoa, which are released into the external environment along with the grass. In the body of the mollusk, a miracidia larva hatches from the parasitic eggs and turns into a sporocyst. Sporocysts reproduce parthenogenetically. From the embryonic cells of the first order sporocyst, second order sporocysts emerge, from which cercariae develop.

Thus, the radiolarian period does not occur in the two-sucking cnidarians. Cercariae actively move and enter the respiratory organs of the mollusks. In the respiratory tract of the mollusk, 100-300 cercariae gather and wrap themselves in a common shell. This collection is called a mucous nodule. Later, these nodules are released into the external environment through the mollusk's spiracle, attaching to plants and other objects. The development of the parasite larvae in the body of the mollusk lasts from 82 days to 6 months. The second intermediate host, ants, eat the mucus nodules containing cercariae, that is, clusters of cysts, and infect them. After 26-62 days in the ant's body, the cercariae transform into metacercariae.

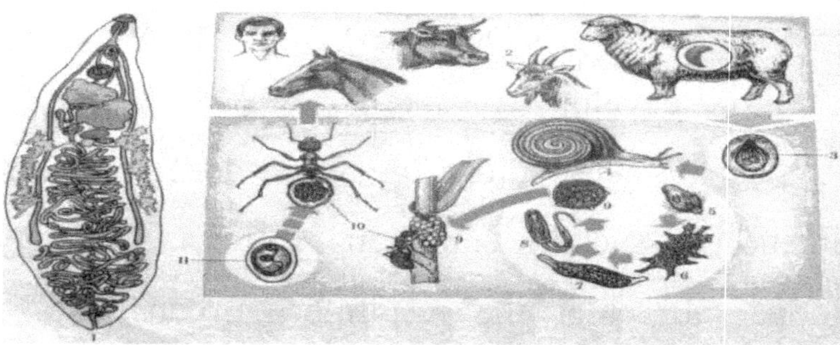

12. Structure and development cycle of the lanceolate sucker – Dicrocoelium lanceolatum:

1-adult form; 2-definitive hosts; 3-egg; 4-first intermediate host and 5-9-larval development; 5-miracidia; 6-7-sporacysts; 8-cercariae; 9-cercarial nodules; 10-second intermediate host; 11-metacercaria.

The definitive hosts infect themselves with parasites by swallowing infected ants along with water and plants. Humans can also be infected in the same way. Metacercariae that have entered the body of the definitive host develop in the liver and bile ducts and reach sexual maturity after 1.5-3 months. The disease caused by the two-sucking tapeworm is called dicroceliosis.

Procedure for conducting work. Examine a stained whole-mount slide of a lancet-shaped insect under a microscope. Find the anterior part of the body where the oral sucker is located in a web.

Also, look at the mouth, esophagus, and two branches of the intestine from the side of the mouth. At the bifurcation of the esophagus is a cirrus sac, and below it is the abdominal sucker. Below the sucker are 2 large, round or oval testes and 1 ovule. Examine the middle of the body and find the small, segmented yolk sacs next to them. The uterus is located in the middle and outer parts of its body, and the eggs in it are visible.

Control and test questions and assignments .

Draw a diagram of the life cycle of the Lancetsimon bivalves in your album and answer the questions below.

1. How does the lancelet dilobite differ from the liver fluke in its structure and development?

2. Which animals are parasitic on which two lancelet worms?

3. How many days does the development of parasite larvae in the body of a mollusk last?

4. How many days does it take for a metacercaria to mature after it has invaded its final host?

5. How many hosts does the Lancet-like two-sucker parasite develop in?

6. In which animal does the metacercariae of the Lancetsimons dicotyledon mature?

7. What is the larval stage before sporacystation called?

8. How do parasitic cercariae differ from radiolarians?

9. How do sporocysts reproduce?

10. What disease does the two suckers of the gnat cause?

Task 3: The structure and development cycle of bloodsuckers.

Type. Other worms - Plathelminthes

Class: Flukes - Trematoda

Category. Schistosomidae - Schistosomatida

Representatives. Schistosoma (Schistosoma mansoni) and Orientobilharzia (Orientobilharzia turkestanica)

Required materials and equipment: Permanently stained slides of bloodsuckers, parasites fixed in alcohol, hand magnifying glasses, microscope, enameled dishes, preparation slides, color tables depicting the structure and development cycle of bloodsuckers.

Objectives of the topic: To study the structure, development cycle, and diseases caused by bloodsuckers.

Summary of the topic. Among the trematodes, schistosomes are considered one of the most dangerous parasites of humans and animals.

Schistosome parasites are blood parasites that live in the veins of the intestines, liver, and bladder of humans and animals. They are mainly distributed in tropical and subtropical countries, namely Africa, Asia, and South America. They are distinguished from other trematodes by their separate sexes. The male's body is quite thick, 15 mmabout 10 cm long, and has a special ovipositor on its abdomen, 20 mmwhere it mates with a long, slender female.

Males have more than 10 testicles, while females have only one oval-shaped ovule.

The suckers of bloodsuckers are poorly developed or absent. Schistosoma lives in the large veins of the abdominal cavity of humans, in the veins of the kidneys and bladder.

Schistosome parasites, or bloodsuckers, are parasitic worms that develop in freshwater mollusks of the genus Planorbis. The female worm eats the walls of human blood vessels and lays eggs in the connective tissue of the bladder wall. As a result, the bladder becomes inflamed and painful. The eggs, which are miracidia larvae, penetrate the intestinal and urinary walls and are then excreted through the host's feces and urine. The miracidia hatch from the eggs, which fall into the water, and enter the body of an intermediate host - a gastropod mollusk. After that, they develop first in the liver of the mollusk, where they develop into mother sporocysts, then daughter sporocysts, radii, and finally cercariae, which have separate tails.

From one miracidium to 200 thousand cercariae develop in a mollusk organism. When the cercariae infect the primary host, that is, a person bathing or in marshes where cercariae are present, the cercariae pierce the host's skin with the help of a stylet, enter the circulatory system, and migrate throughout the organism.

The parasite reaches sexual maturity after 43-55 days and begins to lay eggs (Figure 13). The disease caused by schistosomiasis is called schistosomiasis. According to the World Health Organization, more than 700 million people worldwide suffer from schistosomiasis.

The most common parasites in humans are Schistosoma mansoni, Schistosoma haematobium, and Schistosoma japonisum. In Brazil, more than 4 million people are infected with Schistosoma mansoni, and in Egypt and other Arab countries, 16 million people are infected with Schistosoma haematobium. In some villages in Egypt, 60-95% of the population is infected with this disease.

Schistosoma parasites live in the body of patients for 5-10 years.

Schistosome parasites cause damage to the walls of the bladder, kidneys, and urethra in humans, causing blood to be excreted in the urine. Inflammation of the affected organs and the accumulation of phosphorus salts in the atrophy of the parasite eggs can lead to the formation of stones in the bladder.

In addition, infected people experience itching, symptoms of pneumonia, anemia, diarrhea, and other conditions.

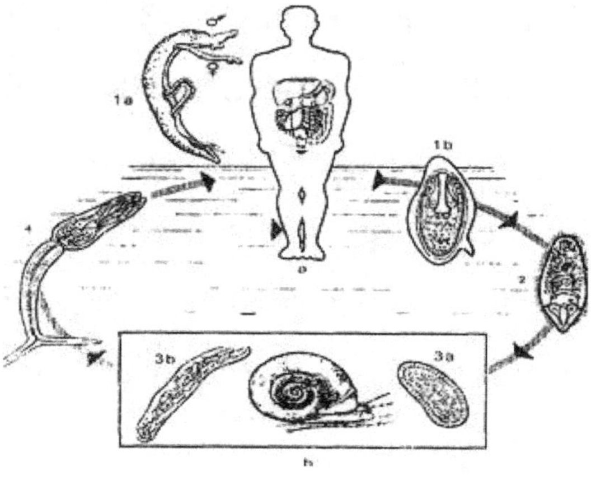

14. Schematic of the development cycle of schistosome (Schistosoma mansoni): *a-primary host; 1a-copulation of female and male parasites; 1b-Sch. mansoni the egg of; 2-miracidium; b-developmental cycle example; 3-mollusk belonging to the genus Planorbis; 3a-first instar sporocyst; 3b-second instar sporocyst; 4-cercariae.*

Another bloodsucker that parasitizes in the intestines, liver, pancreas, and blood vessels of cattle is the Oriental Bilharzia (Orientobilharzia turkestanisa).

Oriental helminthiasis was first discovered in cattle in 1913 by Academician KI Scriabin in Turkestan. This parasite occurs in cattle of all ages and is transmitted mainly through the skin. Infected animals show weakness, diarrhea, blood and fibrinous plaques in their feces, fever, and rapid breathing. The disease caused by the parasite is called oriental helminthiasis. In Uzbekistan, livestock in the Republic of Karakalpakstan and the Khorezm region are mainly affected by the disease.

The Oriental bilgarcia is different from other suckers in that it is bisexual. The male 12,9 mmis 6.4 cm long and has a cuticular tentacle on the ventral side, around which he surrounds the female and lives together. The female is slender and shorter than the male, measuring 4.8 6,8 mmcm in length. The male has a rounded mouth, while the female has a rudimentary mouth. Like other bloodsuckers, it also develops in two hosts. Its intermediate host is freshwater snails and its primary host is cattle. The eggs of oriental tapeworms penetrate the walls of blood vessels and are excreted in the intestines and feces of animals. The eggs contain ready-made larvae -

myracids. The myracids that hatch from the eggs in water find their intermediate hosts - freshwater snails, enter their bodies and develop into sporocysts. The mother sporocyst, in turn, reproduces parthenogenetically, producing 100-200 daughter sporocysts, and each daughter sporocyst produces 100 cercariae, meaning that more than 20,000 cercariae are formed from 1 embryo.

Cercariae develop in the body of mollusks in 18-21 days and emerge from the mollusks into the water. In water, cercariae penetrate the skin of their final hosts, namely cattle. Young parasites migrate to the blood vessels of the liver, stomach, pancreas and pancreas, reach sexual maturity after 2 months and begin to lay eggs again. They can live in the body of the final host for up to 7 years.

15. Orientobilharzia turkestanica
A - The definitive host of the parasite.
B - The intermediate host of the parasite – a freshwater snail.
1. Adult parasite.
2. Egg.
3. Miracidium.
4. Cercaria..

Procedure. After explaining the structure, distribution, developmental cycle, and disease of bloodsuckers, including the orientalis, the students place the orientalis fixed in alcohol in a Petri dish with water and examine it through binoculars or a small microscope objective to distinguish between males and females.

Note that 8 mmthe male is longer than the female (7-) and that the male has a cuticular seta on the ventral side. 12 mmObserve under the microscope that the female has a round body and is slightly smaller than the male (4.8-), and that the male's oral sucker is round, while the female's is not well developed, i.e. the oral sucker is rudimentary.

Control and test questions and assignments .

Draw the life cycle diagrams of Schistosoma and Orientalis in your album and answer the questions below.

1. How long is a female bloodsucker?

2. How many hosts does a bloodsucker develop in?

3. How long does it take for schistosome parasites to reach adulthood after being transmitted to humans?

4. Describe the intermediate hosts of schistosome parasites.

5. What types of schistosome parasites infect humans?

6. How do schistosomes differ from other protozoa in structure and reproduction?

7. How long do schistosome parasites remain in infected people?

8. In which organs of humans do schistosome parasites infect?

9. Which species of bloodsuckers parasitize livestock in Uzbekistan?

10. In which regions of Uzbekistan is the Orientale bacterium most commonly found in livestock?

11. How is the Oriental Reticulum pathogen transmitted to livestock?

12. How long can the Orientobiliary tract pathogen survive in livestock?

5- PRACTICAL TRAINING.

Topic: The structure and development of parasitic unicellular organisms - Dactylogyrhus and Gyrodactylus .

Type. Flatworms - Plathelminthes

Class. Monogenea- Monogenea

Category : Dactylogyridea

Representative . Dactylogirus- Dactylogyrus vastator

Necessary materials and equipment. Permanently stained preparations of Dactylogyrus and Gyrodactylus, microscope, binoculars, magnifying glasses, color charts showing the structure and development cycle of Dactylogyrus and Gyrodactylus.

Objectives of the topic: To study the structure, development cycle, and diseases caused by Dactylogyrhus and Gyrodactylus.

Brief summary of the topic ;

The class Monogeneans includes over 2000 species . They It mainly parasitizes fish, amphibians, reptiles, and some aquatic mammals.

Monogeneans are mainly ectoparasites, with only a few species having undergone a secondary endoparasite transformation.

The body of monogeneans is elongated, flat, leaf-like, and ranges in size from 0.3 mm to 2-3 cm.

The entire life cycle of representatives of monogeneans takes place on a single host. The main characteristic features of animals belonging to this class can be further listed as follows.

The mouthparts are often absent. In addition to the muscular suckers at the posterior end of the body, the attachment organs consisting of hooks and loops are also well developed. Most have eyes. They can sometimes lay one, sometimes several eggs.

The adhesion organs on the head of monogeneans serve to attach the parasite to the host's body while it is feeding. At the posterior end of the body is a more advanced and complex adhesion organ, the disc. Inside the disc are 10 to 16 chitinous loops of various sizes .

Monogeneans develop without an intermediate host, that is, there is no change of host and no reproduction during their life cycle. Usually, two individuals adhere to each other with their genital openings facing outwards and exchange sperm.

The eggs of monogeneans are spherical, oval and filamentous in shape. The fertilized eggs are released into the water . There are also live - bearing species . As a result of the development of the fertilized egg in water , an elongated larva with a ciliary body is formed . The larva moves in water with the help of cilia . At the posterior end of the larva's body there are discs and appendages , and at the anterior end there are eyes, glands and a mouth . They have The nervous and sensory organs are well developed. The further development of the larvae takes place in the host organism , that is, after living a life of free swimming in a certain and hard water, they attach themselves to the body of their host and, having lost their cilia , reach sexual maturity. It should also be noted that the period of maturation of the larvae is not the same in all monogeneans. For example, the larvae of the genus Dactylogyrus reach maturity in 7-9 days and begin to lay eggs . The larvae of the frog 's bladder parasite, the frog 's multi -spined frog, reach sexual maturity after 3 years, like their hosts.

Some species of monogeneans parasitize fish, causing significant damage to fisheries.

Dactylogiruses parasitize in the gills of fish , eating away at the epithelial tissue of the gills . As a result, the fish have difficulty breathing . They stop growing and gaining weight. Many fish die within a few days . Dactylogiruses are 1-3 mm long, they parasitize in the gills of fish and lay eggs there . A ciliated larva hatches from the egg. The larva matures there.

Case 2. Gyrodactylus Systemic role structure and development .

Type . Flatworms – Plathelminthes

Class : Monogenea

Category : Gyrodactylidea

Representative . Gyrodactylus- Gyrodactylus elegans

Another genus of monogeneans, Gyrodactylus elegans, is also a dangerous parasite of fish and causes the disease gyrodactylosis.

Gyrodactylus is biologically very strange . They are also hermaphrodites, with a single testicle and ovary, and live The larva gives birth . Therefore , parasites have constantly developing embryos in their uterus, that is, in the uterus of an adult worm there is only one egg, from which one embryo is formed by parthenogenetic means . Until this embryo reaches adulthood, a second embryo develops inside it , a third embryo inside the second embryo , and a fourth inside the third . All this process takes place in the uterus of the parasite. Thus , the gyrodactylus gives birth to live young, and in this case one parasite gives birth to four young worms .

Gyrodactylus is widespread mainly in Ukraine, Belarus, Uzbekistan and the Krasnodar Territory, causing mass mortality of young fish. The skin of infected fish changes color and spots appear.

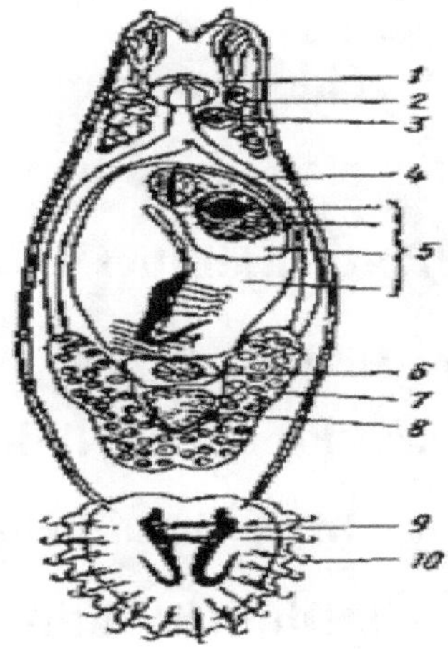

17. Gyrodactylus elegans, a parasite of whales :

1-mouth opening, 2- glands, 3-copulatory organ, 4- intestine, 5- embryos of the four generations, 6- egg, 7- ovary, 8- testis, 9- main loops of the adhesion disc, 10- marginal loops of the adhesion disc.

6 - PRACTICAL TRAINING

Topic: Parasitic unicellular organisms - the structure and developmental stages of the Cerbarian tapeworm, ligula, and echinococcus.

Case 1. The structure and development cycle of the Serbian tapeworm.

Type. Plathelminthes

Class. Cestoda

Category. Pseudophyllidea

Familiy . Diphyllobothridae

And a kil. Diphyllobothrium latum

The purpose of the lesson . To study the structure , development cycle , and motivation of the human body .

Short summary of the topic . The serbart is the longest and largest representative of the serbian , and it is a small intestine of many mammals (dogs , cats , foxes , bears , water bears

, wolves) . The length 15 mof the trunk is 10 cm , and the width is 3-4.5 cm .

The school , that is , the rest of the world , is different from the rest . There are 2 deep holes in the place of the suction cup on the left side of them , which help to close the hole .no such things as science . Germ aphrodisiac proglottids have a genital system similar to that of the male genitalia , but the female genitalia have 3 different organs . One of them is a small hole , and the rest is a small hole and a hole in the spermatic canal .The side of the program is similar to that of the above figure . the front , especially the front o chil a di. Because the width of the joint of the axle is large compared to the length , the name of the parasite is large or wide .A mature articular arb e m o r a l a t i o n comes out to the east .

In this case, the eggs of the tapeworm, which mature in the definitive host, are released into the external environment together with the feces. These eggs develop only in water. After 3-5 weeks, a coracidium, covered with cilia, hatches from the egg. The coracidium is a sharsimone and swims in the water with the help of cilia. Under the ciliated epithelium of the coracidium, there is an oncosphere with 6 loops. The coracidium is swallowed by the cyclops. Inside the cyclops, the coracidium loses its cilia and the oncospheres penetrate the intestinal wall and pass into the body cavity. Here the oncosphere develops into the next larval stage, the procercoid.

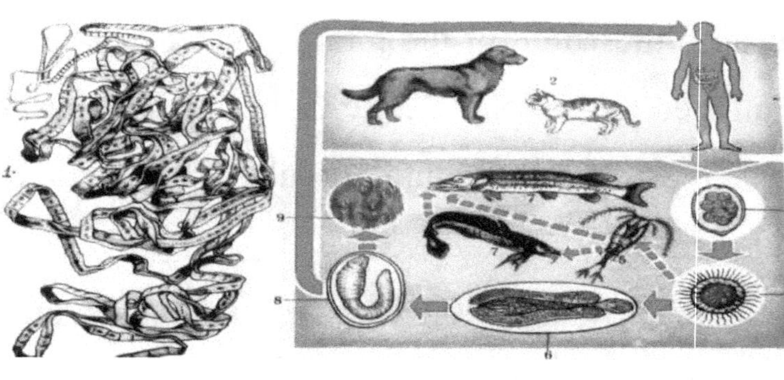

18. Developmental stages of the Cerberus tapeworm (Diphyllobothrium latum): *1- adult Cerberus tapeworm; 2- primary hosts; 3-parasite egg; 4-coracidium larva; 5-first intermediate host-cyclops; 6-procercoid larva; 7-second intermediate host (fish); 8-plerosercoid larva; plerosercoids in fish muscle 9.*

The head of the procercoid has a small, round growth with 6 loops. The development of the procercoid lasts about 3 weeks. Subsequently, the cyclops infected with these larvae is swallowed by carp, smelt and some salmonids. The procercoids pass from the stomach of the fish to the muscles, liver and other organs and develop into the next larval stage - plerosercoid. The plerosercoid 15 mmis 10 mm long and has suckers

- botrya - on its head. This larval stage is considered infectious.

Humans become infected with the Serbian tapeworm when they eat raw or undercooked fish or caviar containing plerosercoid. After 21-36 days, the plerosercoid 20 mdevelops into a sexually mature broad tapeworm 8-15, sometimes longer, in the human body.

In addition to the main host and two intermediate hosts, in some cases a reservoir host may also participate in the development of this parasite. Such reservoir hosts are various predatory fish, which devour small fish infected with plerocercoids. In these small fish, the plerocercoids settle in the muscles and other organs of the predatory fish and maintain their viability. For example, a single quart of fish has been found to contain up to 250 plerocercoids. In one day or night, an infected person or animal can shed up to 21 million parasitic eggs.

The disease caused by the Serbian tapeworm is called diphyllobothriasis. This parasite can live in the human intestine for up to 15 years or more. Because they are large, they eat a lot of food. People infected with diphyllobothriasis experience headaches and dizziness, growth and development delays, decreased performance, changes in bowel habits, weakness, decreased appetite, and fatigue. The amount of hemoglobin and erythrocytes in a person decreases, which leads to anemia.

The Serbian tapeworm is widespread in areas where the population of river and lake shores feeds mainly on fish (it causes great harm to the population and predators living in Karelia, the St. Petersburg region, the Baltic coast, Siberia, the atrophy of the Irtysh, Ob, Lena, Yenisei,

Amur, Neva, Volga river basins, and the atrophy of Lake Baikal).

Comprehensive measures are being taken to combat diphyllobothriasis. Measures are being taken, including treating sick people, preventing the contamination of water bodies, and avoiding the consumption of spoiled fish, namely poorly salted and freshly frozen fish. Sick people are treated with fennel or pumpkin seeds.

Procedure. Examine the head of a tapeworm with a wide, painted tape attached to the sides of the scolex through a small objective of a microscope. Find the cracks - botrya. Look closely at the neck of the head, where it is attached to the body.

Examine the preparation of a mature segment of the Serbian tapeworm. Note the width of the segment. It is much larger than its length, and also note the clearly visible flower-like uterus.

On the anterior side of the segment lie the dark whorls of the flower-like uterus. In this part of the proglottid, find the light, round cirrus sac between the two whorls of the uterus. Small ovules are located near the lateral border of the joint. Slightly inward from the edge of the joint, above the ovules, lie the seeds.

A two-jointed ovule is visible near the bottom of the proglottid.

Control and test questions and assignments.

Draw the scolex, hermaphrodite, and adult segments of the Serbian tapeworm, as well as the developmental cycle, in your album, and answer the questions below.

1. How does the Serbian tapeworm differ from other tapeworms in terms of its structure and development cycle?

2. How many hosts does the Serbian tapeworm develop on?
3. Why is the tapeworm called a tapeworm?
4. How does the genitalia of the Serbian tapeworm differ from that of the cattle tapeworm?
5. How many eggs and sperm does a tapeworm have in each segment?
6. What are the larval stages in the development of the Serbian tapeworm?
7. How long does it take for the plerosercoid larva of the parasite to reach sexual maturity after being transmitted to humans?
8. What disease does the Serbian tapeworm cause?
9. How long can the Serbian tapeworm live in the human body?
10. Tell me the number of segments and length of the Serbian tapeworm.

Case 2. The structure and development cycle of echinococcus.

Type. Plathelminthes

Class. Cestoda

Category. - Cyclophyllide a

Family.– Teniidae

And a kil. Echinococcus granulosus

In the case of nexinococci and its preparations fixed in alcohol , freshly slaughtered sheep , the lungs and liver of the chicken are removed from the nexinococci cysts , the exinococci scol e x and Arthritis preparation , paint preparations , microscopes , loupes , instruments and tools , clamps , enamel , preparation , exogenousstructure

The purpose of the lesson . Study the structure of the exhaust gas , the engine cycle and the efficiency of the engine .

Short summary of the topic . The price is 28-40 days . It 's a good science .The first and second joints of the scoliosis are germ fronds , and there are about 50 seeds , spermatozoa , genital bursa , ovule , melisth , and ovule .400-800 t eggs are filled in each joint of the axis .It can live up to 6 months , sometimes up to 1 year , inside meat and other meat containers .The front and rear joints of the exhaust pipe are the same as the main shaft . It emerges from this joint and passes through a 5-25 cm thick layer and lays its eggs on other plants .

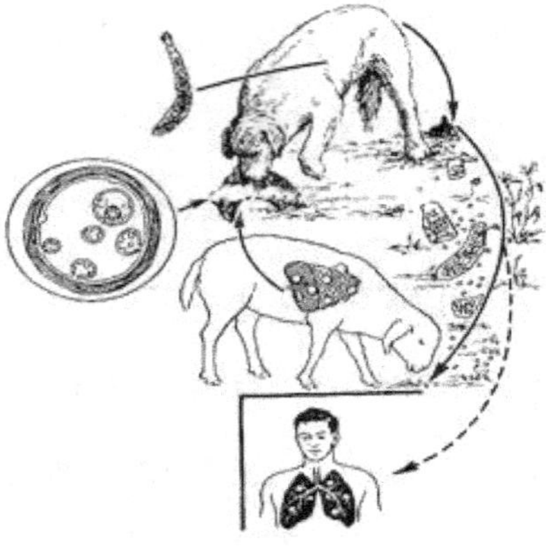

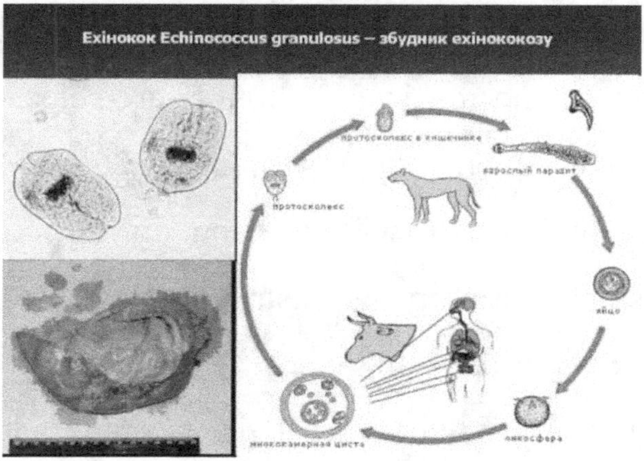

19th cent . Development cycle scheme of Echinococcus granulosus .

Middle - aged animals - sheep , goats , camels , and other grasses - are infected with the virus .

. The cysts of exogenous cocci can grow for 10-30 years .Inside the puff , there is an ex - inoculate larva , and the main part of it is reduced to the inside of the stomach .

If the dog eats the liver of the dog , the larvae of the rex in 2-3 months are released into the environment . begins to produce eggs .

It is also widely used in agriculture , livestock farming (Austria , New Zealand , several regions of North Africa , and many countries in Asia) . It is a combination of humanity and humanity .Humans can infect themselves with Echinococcal eggs when they come close to dogs , touch them , eat other meat - eating animals , and rub their skin .di. Because the hair of the dog has a lot of small eggs .That 's why everyone should follow the rules .

The liver is damaged , the lungs are damaged , and breathing difficulties are reported .

In order to prevent the damage of the dogs in the fight against the echinococcosis , it is important to know the importance of the language . In order to prevent the infection of dogs with ecchinococcal larvae , it is mandatory to remove all live animals or dead animals from the vet .my With the bubble level of the exogenous organ , the organ tissue is sent to the ex nic utilization center , and the remaining part of the animal 's body is used for the organ tissue recovery .work a language a di. If the skeletal muscles or internal organs of the animal are in a strong state of exogenous exudate , they are used as a complement .Echinococcosis is mainly treated by immunological methods .

Procedure for conducting work . Observe the total microstructure of the exudate through the small objective of the microscope . Get to the heart of the parasite . Close the sko l e ksd a dig a n 4 t a sucker v a Find out about the science of kha rtumch a sid a . Count the number of programs . Please copy the first and fourth programs .Place the liver and lungs of sheep or goats prepared with exudate in an enamel container with water . Look behind you and find the second girl inside the bubble .

Control and test questions and assignments.

Draw a diagram of the development cycle of Echinococcus in your album and answer the questions below.

1. Who does Echinococcus infect and how long does it last?
2. How many parts is the body of an adult echinococcus divided into, and what organs are located in its scolex?
3. How many eggs are in a mature Echinococcus cyst?
4. How long can adult echinococcus survive in its definitive host?

5. Who are the intermediate hosts of Echinococcus and in which organs does it parasitize?

7-PRACTICAL TRAINING.

Topic : Parasitic unicellular organisms - the structure and development of cattle and pig tapeworms and pinworms .

Case 1. The structure and development cycle of the cattle tapeworm.

Type. Other worms - Plathelminthes

Class: Tapeworms – Cestoda

Category: Tapeworms - Cyclophyllidae

Family. Teniidae

Representative. Cattle tapeworm - Taeniarhynchus saginatus

Required materials and equipment. Wet preparations of the cattle tapeworm fixed in alcohol, micropreparations of the head, hermaphrodite and mature joints of the cattle tapeworm, color tables depicting the development and structure of the cattle tapeworm, magnifying glass, microscope, slides, Petri dishes, pieces of finned meat fixed in alcohol.

Objectives of the topic: To get acquainted with the structure, signs of adaptation to parasitism, and development cycle of the cattle tapeworm, a tapeworm.

Brief content of the topic. The adult cattle tapeworm mainly infects the small intestine of humans. The body of the parasite is about 4 10 mcm long and 2 14 mmcm wide. The body consists of a head (scolex), a neck and about a thousand proglottids.

The scolex has 4 suckers. Between the suckers there is a rudimentary sac, which does not have chitinous loops. Therefore, the cattle tapeworm is also called an unarmed tapeworm.

The genitals appear from about the 200th joint. In hermaphrodite joints, male and female genitals mature first.

The number of seeds in each proglottid is about 1000, and each ovule is bifurcated. The mature joints at the end of the body have a gynoecium and 18-35 outgrowths growing from the main gynoecium to the sides.

These growths, in turn, branch out and cover the entire surface of the proglottid. The last mature proglottid is 16 mm long 20 mmand 4 mm wide 7 mm, and they emerge singly from the strobila.

The larval stage of the cattle tapeworm, the cysticercus, also lives as a parasite. The cysticercus is oval in shape, about the size of a pea. Inside it are scolexes with 4 suckers. The cysticercus lives in the meat of cattle and is called a finna.

Thus, cattle tapeworm is a biohelminth, and humans are the primary hosts of this parasite, with cattle, zebu, buffalo, and jackals as intermediate hosts (Figure 15).

People are mainly infected with this parasite by eating raw, undercooked or undercooked beef. The shell of the cysticercus that enters the human body is dissolved by gastric juice and bile, and the larvae that emerge from it attach to the intestinal wall with their suckers and begin to develop, reaching sexual maturity after 2-3 months.

The last mature cilia break off from the mite and are expelled. It can live in the human body for 18-20 years or more, laying up to 600 million eggs per year, or 11 billion eggs over its lifetime. Cattle ingest the parasite's eggs through food, water, and sometimes human feces.

In the stomach of cattle, the shell of the parasite egg dissolves under the influence of juices, and the larva that emerges from it - the oncosphere - penetrates the walls of the stomach or intestines with the help of loops, passes into the blood vessels, spreads to the body with the blood and settles in the skeletal muscles, tongue, heart, eyes, brain, and other organs. After a certain time, that is, after 4-6 months, it turns into a pea-sized bubble. This period is called finna, and the disease it causes is called finniosis.

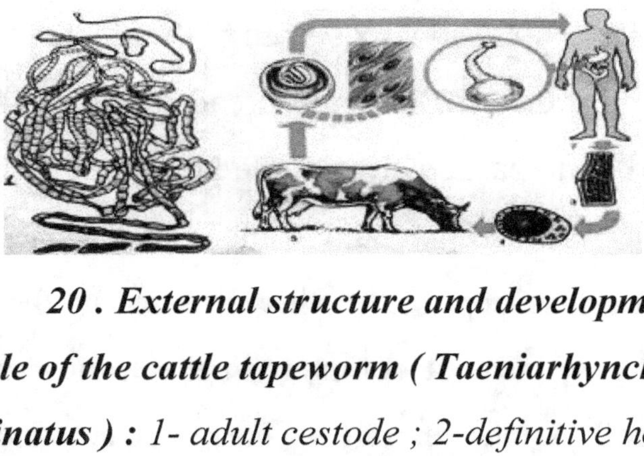

20 . External structure and development cycle of the cattle tapeworm (Taeniarhynchus saginatus) : *1- adult cestode ; 2-definitive host ; 3-mobile segment; 4-egg with oncosphere; 5-intermediate host; 6-finna (cysticercus); 7-development of cestode in the intestine of the*

definitive host ; 8-meat of an animal infected with cysticercus .

In general, the sexually mature stage of the cattle tapeworm is called taeniarhynchus (Taeniarhynchus saginatus) and the disease it causes is called taeniarhynchosis. The disease caused by the larval stage (Cysticercus bovis) is called cysticercosis. It is clear from this that people infected with taeniarhynchus and cattle infected with cysticercosis are both infected.

Tapeworm is widespread throughout the world. In particular, people in Africa, South America, Australia, and some countries in Asia are most susceptible to this disease. In the CIS, tapeworm is most common in the Caucasus, the Central Asian republics, Kazakhstan, and the northern regions of Russia. In Uzbekistan, this disease is most common among the population of the Khorezm region and the Republic of

Karakalpakstan. The main reason for this is the widespread consumption of the national dish "ijjan" made from minced beef among the local population.

It has also been partially recorded in the Bukhara and Samarkand regions. Cysticercosis occurs in cattle and causes significant economic damage to livestock farming. Because the price of meat infected with cysticercosis is low. Such meat can only be consumed after disinfection.

Cattle are particularly susceptible to cysticercosis, especially in private households. This is because some households do not have toilets, and even if they do, they do not meet sanitary standards. Cattle meat must undergo veterinary inspection in poultry houses. Raw or undercooked cattle meat should not be eaten, and raw minced meat should not be tasted. In addition, it is necessary to build closed toilets in each apartment and keep them clean.

Exercise method. Place the cattle tapeworm in an enameled water bath and observe its external structure, namely its flat, tapeworm-like body, its segmentation, its head, and the presence of an unsegmented neck, using a magnifying glass. Examine the head of a tapeworm under a microscope to find its suckers, and observe the organs inside the immature and mature segments. Distinguish between a hermaphrodite segment and a mature segment. Observe the eggs inside the mature segments.

Control and test questions and assignments.

Draw a diagram of the structure and life cycle of the cattle tapeworm in your album and answer the questions below.

1. Who is infected with the cattle tapeworm?

2. How long is a cattle tapeworm?

3. How does cattle tapeworm differ in structure from swine tapeworm?

4. How many hosts does the cattle tapeworm develop on?

5. What disease does cattle tapeworm cause in humans?

Case 2. The structure and development cycle of the pork tapeworm.

Type. Other worms - Plathelminthes

Class: Tapeworms - Cestoda

Category. Tapeworms - Cyclophyllidea

Family. Teniidae

Representative. Pig tapeworm - Taenia solium

Required materials and equipment. Alcohol-fixed wet preparations of pork tapeworm, micropreparations of scolex, hermaphrodite and adult joints, microscope, enameled cuvette, preparation slides, color tables depicting the structure and development cycle of pork tapeworm.

Objective: To study the structure, development cycle, and disease caused by the pork tapeworm.

Brief content of the topic. The adult stage of the pork tapeworm is parasitic in the small intestine of a person. It is 1.5- 3 m, sometimes 5 mup to a meter long, and has a head, that is, a scolex, a neck and about 900 proglottids. The head has 4 suckers and two rows of chitinous hooks of various sizes on the proboscis. The pig tapeworm is also called an armed tapeworm due to the presence of hooks. Each of the pig tapeworm proglottids contains hundreds of gametes and a single, three-lobed ovule (Figure 16).

The uterus of this worm differs from that of the cattle tapeworm in that it has 7-12 lateral branches and is constantly filled with eggs. The last mature proglottids are 10 mm long 12 mmand 5 mmatrophied in width. In addition, the mature segments of the pig tapeworm are suddenly separated from the strobila by 5-7 segments and are excreted with the host's feces, and these segments are immobile. The larva is called a cysticercus. This larva parasitizes in various tissues and organs, wrapped in a special shell. The cysticercus is a pea-sized bubble filled with a clear liquid. At its tip are 4 suckers and a scolex covered with hooks.

The main host of the pork tapeworm is humans. The adult tapeworm parasitizes in the human small intestine. Pigs, dogs, cats, and camels are considered intermediate hosts of this parasite. In this case, pigs and the above-mentioned animals are infected with the eggs of the worms through water and various foods. The 6-looped larva (oncosphere) that hatches from the egg in the body of the intermediate host travels through the blood and lymphatic vessels, settles in the muscle tissue, brain, eyes, and other organs, wraps itself in a special shell, and after 2-4 months turns into the second larval stage - cysticercus.

Cysticercosis can live in the body of a pig for 3 to 6 years. Cysticercosis is also called finworm. People become infected with the pork tapeworm by eating undercooked pork meat that is infected with cysticercosis. The disease caused by the adult form of the pork tapeworm is called taeniasis, and the disease caused by the larval stage is called cysticercosis. People can get both taeniasis and cysticercosis.

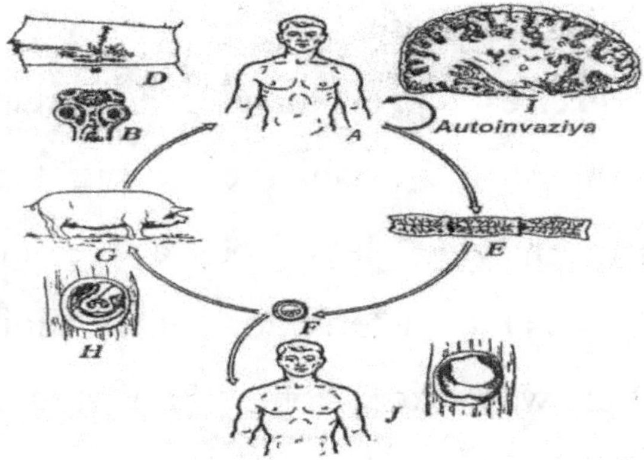

Figure 21. Life cycle of the pork tapeworm: *A-primary host - man, B-head part, l)-hermaphrodite joint, E-group of mature joints, F-egg, G-intermediate host, H-flesh in meat, l-fins in the human brain, J-man as a facultative intermediate host.*

Only pigs are infected with cysticercosis. Porcine cysticercosis is found in the CIS, in particular in Ukraine, Belarus, Azerbaijan and some regions of Russia. The main source of the spread of this disease is considered to be people with tapeworm disease.

Exercise procedure. Examine the preparation of the strobila of a pig tapeworm under a magnifying glass. Look at the surface of the joints and determine which joint the preparation was taken from. Make sure that the body is flat and not twisted.

Note that the pig tapeworm has two rows of hooks on its scolex, which is a single row of suckers at the head, unlike the cattle tapeworm, which has four suckers and two rows of hooks. Examine a stained slide of a hermaphroditic proglottid of a pig tapeworm under a small microscope objective and identify the seminiferous tubule, yolk sac, melisma, and ovary.

Control and test questions and assignments.

Draw a picture of the structure and development cycle of the pork tapeworm in your album and answer the questions below.

1. Who does the adult pork tapeworm infect?
2. How long is the pig tapeworm and how does it differ from the cattle tapeworm in terms of structure and reproduction?
3. How many hosts does the pork tapeworm develop in and what disease does it cause in humans?
4. How is pork tapeworm transmitted to humans?
5. How many segments does the uterus of a mature pig tapeworm have?

6. What animals are the intermediate hosts of the pork tapeworm?

7. In which countries is the pig tapeworm most prevalent?

8. How are the mature segments of the pork tapeworm excreted?

8-PRACTICAL TRAINING

Topic: Parasitic nematodes - Human roundworm, pinworm, and tapeworm structure and development stages

Case 1. The structure and development cycle of human ascariasis.

Type. True worms -Nemathelminthes

Class. N e mNematoda

Category. Ascarid

And a kil. Ascaris lumbricoides

Required materials and equipment. Make a fixation with 4-6 % formalin solution on scar tissue , cross - sectional wire microscope , microscope , gloves , small needles , surgical knives , forceps r , preparation , entomology , bottom wax and wax , and the outer and inner structure of the ascarid , as well as the life cycle are shown .

The purpose of the lesson . To study the characteristics of the structure and structure of the model , the development cycle and the driving force .

Short summary of the topic . The body of the human skull is narrow , the front and back ends are narrow , and the cross section is straight.

The body of the Ascarid is covered with a multi - layered cuticle , and because of its semiconducting properties , the body is in constant state . Hypodermic skin over the cuticle . It is a strong muscle that stretches along the length of the hypodermic muscle .

Ascarids are semi - sexual and the genitals are long and slender . The genital glands of the female are paired , the front thin ends of the tube are the ovaries , and the slightly wider part of it forms the oviduct . The rhombus expands and forms a pair of cells , joining each other and exiting with a sexual hole in the middle of the body . What is the meaning of the word.

The male reproductive system consists of a penis , the thin end of which is the testicles , and the thick part serves as the spermatic cord . The spermatic cord is located in the vagina , passes into the ejaculatory duct , and then into the cloaca . o chil a di. There are two spicules inside the cuticle , that is , there is a joining organ .

Inside the guide A person with scabies feels like he is infected with a parasite .

A single female scorpion lays 200-250 thousand eggs in one day and night . The seed of Ascarid has three layers of skin , but this newly laid seed is very useful . In order for it to have the ability to hatch , it should be 15-25 days out of the hatch .

The external environment A student can keep the privilege of living for up to 10 years. If there is a larva in the stomach , the egg can be infected by consuming unboiled water , unwashed vegetables , strawberries , strawberries , and other foods that have been left on the surface .

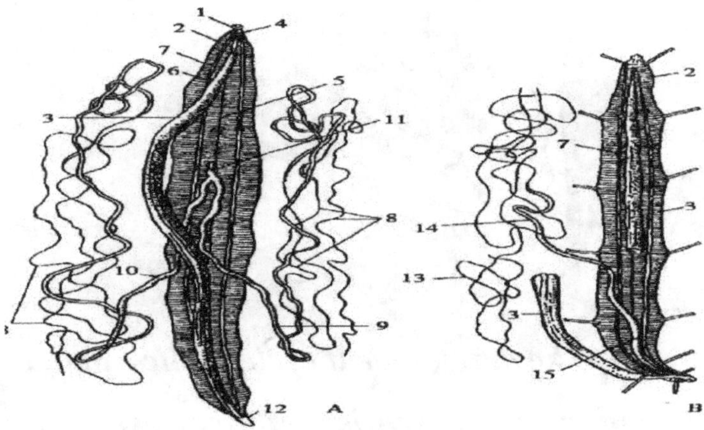

22. Internal structure of Ascaris: A-female. B-male: *1-lips, 2-esophagus, 3-intestine, 4-laryngeal nerve ring, 5-abdominal nerve, 6-excretory system tube, 7-phagocytic cells, 8-ovary, 9-oviduct, 10-uterus, 11-vagina, 12-anal opening, 13-testicle, 14-vas deferens, 15-vas deferens.*

After the egg falls into the stomach , the membrane of the egg dissolves under the action of gastric juices , the larva passes into the blood from the intestine , migrates to the liver , heart , and lungs for 10 days . a di.

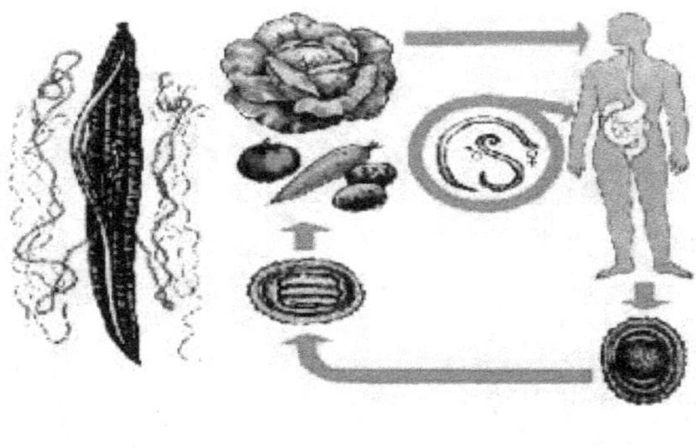

23. The development cycle of the human roundworm (Ascaris lumbricoides).

You can learn by showing . Make a solution of 4-6 % form of solution for pigs Hold one or two of the ascarids with a pair of clamps , put them in water , and with the help of a hand loupe , look at the structure of the skin .Ask for help Try to squeeze the body with your hands and try to bend it and make it as elastic as possible .Pay attention to the fact that the back of the scorpion is dark in color , the body is in the same shape , there are no joints and attachment organs , and the front and rear ends are thin .Find the mouth of the front three and the three muscles of its atrophy . Describe the difference between male and female scorpions in external appearance If the scorpion is alive , before cutting its cuticle crosswise , water is poured into it and it is cut under water , otherwise its body liquid will come out and cover the eye . It can burn organs . Next , with the left hand , the scar is removed and the bottom of the head is pressed , and with the right hand , the cuticle of the upper part of the head is cut .The cuticle is cut long and tightly , and the hair is tightly folded .Help me with my hand In order to make it easy to observe the internal organs of the ascarid , the free part of the right muscles should be bent to the right .Find the hypodermic side of the open scar , and reach the side of the tear duct . The diameter of the cavity of the penis is divided into the sex system .With the help of the preparation , raise them to the surface of the water and , depending on the increase in the diameter of the cells , remove the eggs , the egg ducts , etc.a niql a ng. Make sure that the two children join together to make a coin . Pay attention to the structure of the intestine before sexual intercourse .Observe the micro section of the ascarid through the small objective of the microscope . Find the internal diameter of the atrial cavity of the ascarid

, it is visible in a flat , sometimes flat shape . It is possible to see several reproductive systems in the form of internal organs . There are a few things that can be done in the case of Ascarid . The smallest embryo , filled with cells , is an embryo . One end of them is in the middle of the ovary , and the other end is in the middle part of the uterus . see a di.

To see the multi - layered cuticle of Ascarid and its overlying hypodermic , cross - sectional view of the microscope Observe through the objective lens and draw a picture of it . In order to study the shape , structure and size of the Ascaris egg , cut a small piece from the part near the vagina , place it on an object or a piece of paper , put a drop of water on it and crush it with a glass rod . Observe the prepared preparation through the small objective lens of the microscope .

Control and test questions and assignments.

The structure of the male and female sperm , cross - sectional images , and the pig Draw the flow cycle diagram of the ask arid on paper . Please click below .

1. What is the length of a person 's body ?
2. What is the organ of the cuticle of the scalp ?
3. Explain the developmental cycle of Ascaris .
4. How many eggs does a female spider lay in a day ?
5. Ascarid eggs can survive in the environment for how long ?
6. What is the infectious situation in the external environment of Ascarid Tuxum

Case 2. The structure and development cycle of children 's dreams .

Type. True worms - Nemathelminthes

Class. N e m a t o d a l a r - Nematoda

Category. Oxyurid a l a r - Oxyurida

And a kil. Roundworm - Enterobius vermicularis

Required materials and equipment 4-6 % form lind fixed bulb , microscope , microscope , tool and tool holder , gloves and clamps . The structure and growth cycle of all types of gyjj are shown in two sections .

The purpose of the lesson is to study the structure , development cycle , and motivation of children 's brains .

Brief content of the lesson . A sharp - tailed nemesis or a ball - shaped snake is very common . that is, the length of the female is 10-

12 mm, the length of the male is 2- 5 mm(21 cm)

.

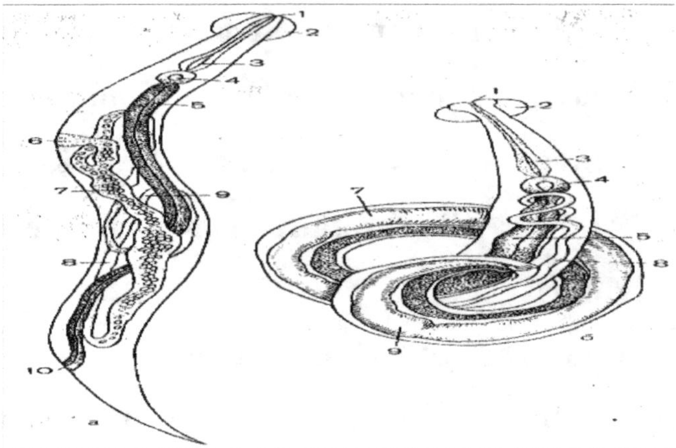

24- Round worm (Enterobius vermicularis) : *a - female **;** b-erk a gi; 1- o gzi; 2-v e zikul a'osimt a si ; 3-red a chi; 4th bulb; 5-ort a ich a gi; 6th sexual organ ; 7-9 is a part of the reproductive system ; 10th floor door .*

b

Because of the sharp a ailed nematode , the body of the female is narrower and sharper than the tip of the tail . The end of a man 's sleeve is spir a lsim o n bur a lg a n. The first part of the body is covered with cuticles and cuticles .It is the presence of a single spicule in the ascarid of the male .He has three mouths .The esophagus is filled with bulbus .Bulbusd a cuticle with ch a yn a sh pl a stink a l a ri o r .

It affects the second half of the small intestine and the large intestine , especially in young children . Before laying the eggs , the liquid is secreted .This liquid helps to seal the egg .The parasite gets out of the anal opening and releases its own liquid , and the mechanical and toxic - allergic effects of egg - laying , itch the peri - anal organs .The results are very good .The female mosquito dies after laying eggs . The eggs become infective within 4-6 hours . The female of this parasite lives for 25-30 days . The male kills the female by incubating it .

In some cases , the parasite Enterobius parasite leads to the formation of dysbacteriosis , that is , to a disruption of the normal intestinal microflora . olib kel adi , this is the same vb a tid , intestinal function disorders and the development of intestinal inflammation , acute intestinal infectious diseases , etc. a pp e ndisid kha vfini o shir a di. In other cases , the eggs get inside the underwear , between the fingers and nails , and if the child does not wash his hands properly , the eggs get into the child 's stomach . Therefore , it can be used for several years within a year .

In order to fight against gyjj , the healers ordered to do an enema with hot water and a solution of natural soap , but this did not give good results . Vonkin , komba ntrin , v e rm o x , pip e r azin , m e d a min , a dipin a tk a bi d o ril a r hand to use gijj a bil a nk a s a ll a ng a nb e m o rl a rni .

To prevent enterobiasis , children should be taught to observe strict personal hygiene rules from a young age . Children should be taught to keep their nails trimmed and their clothes ironed . To reduce diarrhea , children should drink half a glass of red carrot juice twice a day for 2-3 weeks .

In general , there are about 20 species of sharp - tailed nematodes . CIS d a It 's the kind of thing that 's going to happen .

The order of conducting the activity . Fix with 4-6 % formalin solution and place the bulb in a glass or Petri dish with water and cover the external view with a magnifying glass or binoculars . Observe the differences in the structure of the male and female , as well as the size of the male and female . The internal structure of the nematode can be seen with a small objective of the microscope Learn by watching .

Control and test questions and assignments.

The structure of the feeding and reproductive systems of the female and male parrots Just smell it .

Draw the structure of each of them on paper and write them down .

1. Explain the systematic state of children 's sleep .

2. Tell me that the length of the female and the male of each uterus is different in the body .

3. How does the structure and growth of children 's teeth differ from that of a normal person ?

4. How many eggs do children lay at night ?

5. How long does it take for children to become contagious after they have been exposed to chickenpox ?

6. How long did the female of all of these birds live ?

7. What is the meaning of the language of the world ?

Case 3. Relationship structure and development cycle.

Type. Roundworms – Nemathelminthes

Class: Nematoda

Family. Spirurids – Spirurida

Representative. Rishta - Dracunculus medinensis

Required materials and equipment. 4-6% formalin Fixed bond, loupes, tables reflecting the bond's structure and development cycle.

Objective of the topic: To study the structure of the bond, its development cycle, and the disease that causes it.

Brief content of the topic. The tapeworm (Dracunculus medinensis) or dracunculus is a thread-like nematode, known in the Central Asian republics as rishta (thread). The thinker Abu Ali ibn Sino is the first to call the tapeworm irkalmedini and to study the disease caused by the parasite.

The species is unisexual, with marked sexual dimorphism. The female can range in length from 32 cm to 150 cm, while the male 30 mmis only 12 cm long (Fig. 24).

The parasite is a biohelminth, and 2 hosts participate in the development cycle. The primary host of the parasite is a person, and in some cases, monkeys, dogs, cats, foxes, raccoons, leopards and other mammals. The sexually mature parasite lives as a parasite in the connective tissue under the skin of its primary hosts, and often under the skin of the feet. The intermediate host is a small aquatic crustacean - cyclops. The male of the worm dies after insemination of the female. After the female of the worm is fertilized, it moves under the skin of the human's arms and legs to give birth to larvae, and after a certain time, swellings appear on the skin. Such swellings burst when they come into contact with water (when washing hands and feet or bathing), and the parasite's larvae fall into the water from them.

In water, the hookworm larvae are ingested by the cyclops as food. The larvae develop in the cyclops' body and become infective (infested) after 12-14 days. Humans and other primary hosts ingest the infected cyclops through water and transmit the hookworm to themselves.

In the intestine of the primary host, the cyclops is digested under the influence of digestive secretions, and the larvae that emerge from it pass through the intestinal wall into the circulatory system and migrate throughout the organism.

After the migration period is over, the larva of the hookworm settles in the subcutaneous fat layer of the patient and reaches sexual maturity after a year, that is , 8-12 months after the person is bitten, reddish blisters appear on the skin, especially on the skin of the feet, and these blisters burst. After that, the female hookworms migrate back under the skin and repeat the life cycle described above.

More than 15 species of Cyclops worldwide are considered intermediate hosts of the parasite. Only 5 species of Cyclops have been identified in the CIS as intermediate hosts of the parasite. The disease caused by the parasite is called dracunculiasis. If the tick dies under the skin of an infected person, the parasite's toxic substances are absorbed into the human body, resulting in various rashes (such as scaly skin) on the body, itching, dizziness, difficulty breathing, and weight loss. Sometimes, inflammation of the joints, nausea, and vomiting also occur. This disease is widespread mainly in countries with a warm climate, namely in Africa, Latin America and South Asia, as well as in Iran, Iraq, Afghanistan, and the Middle East. In Central Asia, ringworm was first discovered in Bukhara by A.P. Fedchenko in 1872, and Professor A.M. Isayev fully studied the development cycle of ringworm and developed measures to eliminate it. Currently, the Rishta is not practiced in our republic. In 1932, the Rishta was completely abolished in the former Soviet Union. The main reasons for the abolition of the Rishta were the drying or disinfection of the reservoirs that were its source, the construction of water pipelines, the prohibition of drinking raw water from reservoirs, the prohibition of washing hands and feet in water bodies used for drinking, and the identification and treatment of people with Rishta.

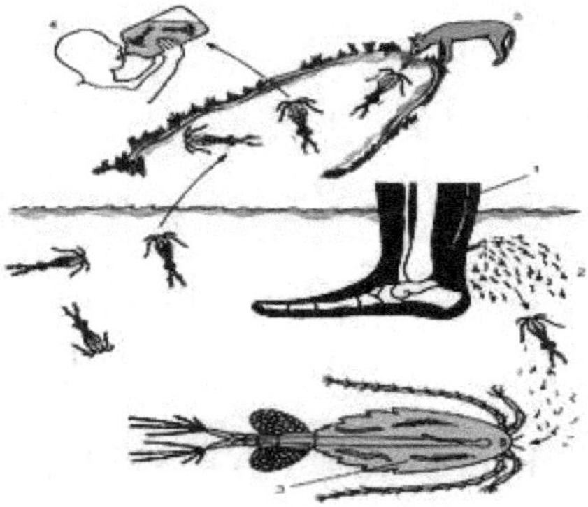

25 . Dracunculus medinensis (** *Dracunculus* **medinensis) development cycle scheme :** *1-* ***basic *Host - sexually mature hookworm parasitic under human skin; 2-hookworm larvae falling from a human body into the water , 3 - a cyclops infected with hookworm larvae , 4.5 - a person and a dog*

swallowing a hookworm infected with hookworm larvae with water .

Control and test questions and assignments.

Draw a diagram of the relationship development cycle in your album and answer the questions below.

1. How long are the female and male of the chain, and who do they parasitize?
2. How many masters does the development cycle of a relationship take?
3. What organs does the sexually mature hookworm infect?
4. Who are the intermediate masters of the relationship and how are they harmed?
5. How long do the larvae of the worm become infective in the intermediate host?
6. How is rabies transmitted to humans and what diseases does it cause?

7. How long does it take for the primary host organism to reach sexual maturity?

8. How many Cyclops rings are considered intermediate masters of the ring, which are located in the world and the CIS?

9. What are the symptoms of people who have been hurt by a relationship?

10.In which countries are people most affected by the coronavirus?

11.Who first discovered the bond in Central Asia, when and in which region, and who studied the development cycle?

9-PRACTICAL TRAINING.

Topic: Parasitic unicellular organisms - the structure of roundworms, hookworms, and trichinella.

Case 1. The structure and development cycle of the roundworm nematode.

Type. True worms - Nemathelminthes

Class. N e m a t o d a - Nematoda

Category. Trichos phalid a - Trichoc e phalida

And keel. A human - made animal - Trichoc e phalus trichiurus

Required materials and equipment.4-6 % form a lind a fixation of male and female trichocephalus , structure and growth cycle of trichocephalus are shown on wall , microscope , glass and glass , preparation

The purpose of the lesson . To study the structure , development cycle and drive efficiency of the electric motor .

Short summary of the topic . It is as thin as the first part of the machine , and it is easy to get to the back part (Fig . 22) .

He was the main guide of the people of the city . It is semi - sexed, the length of the male is

30- 40 mm, and the back He made a big part of it with the help of his own house .The seeds of nematodes come out of the soil of the house .

People are exposed to the disease by eating unwashed fruits and vegetables and ingesting the infectious eggs of the nematode . This is what happened in one month . He lived for 5 years . It 's a good place to be with a child .One female lays 1,000 to 3,500 eggs per day .It is easy to get infected after 20-30 days .

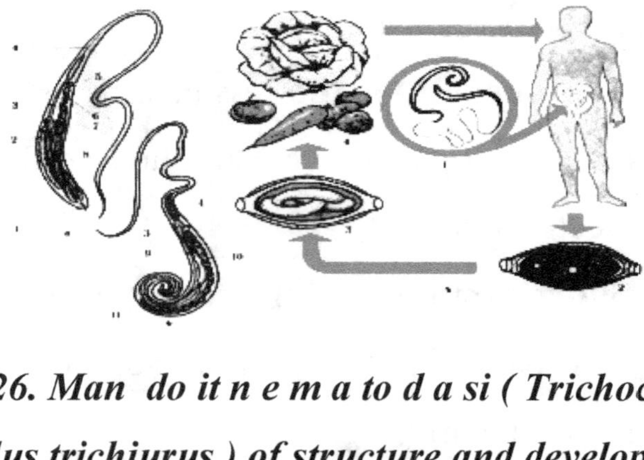

26. Man do it n e m a to d a si (Trichoc e phalus trichiurus) of structure and development cycle : *a - female , b - male a gi : 1- anal hole , 2- egg 3- intestine , 4- esophagus , 5- sexual opening*

, 6- vagina , 7- uterus , 8- ovary , 9- vas deferens , 10- seminal vesicle , 11- seminal vesicle : ***v - od a m do it nematode development cyclical Scheme :***

1- in the organism adult mature parasite , 2 - seeded egg , 3- infectious in the state egg (inside) mature larva with), for 4 people infection factors

..

Pig - Trichocephalus suis , cow - Trichocephalus ovis , q o r a m o ll a rd a - Trichocephalus scribble type parasitism Do it .

The work to pass methodology .

Your body head by topping and in the eyes Please come . A man . and a woman nematodes tail towards he/ she /it to be in love with each other possible .

Control and test questions and assignments.

Draw a picture of the old machine on a sheet of paper and write it down .

1. Monitoring the system status of the computer .
2. What is the difference between the length of the body and the body ?
3. How many eggs does a roundworm lay in a day and how long does it take for the eggs to become infectious under favorable conditions ?
4. How do you feel about having sex with a pregnant woman ?
5. It 's a good idea How long did he live in this world ?
6. What is the best way to prepare for the development of new products ?
7. What kinds of things are different in different countries ?

Case 2. Structure and development cycle of the roundworm nematode .

Type. True worms - Nemathelminthes

Class. N e m a t o d a l a r - Nematoda

Category. R a bditid a l a r - in Rhabditi

Family. A nkiloct o m a tid a l a r - Ancylostomatida

And a kil. Ancylostoma duodenale - Ancylostoma duodenale

Required materials and equipment.. Prepared dye micrographs of male and female oblique nematodes and the structure of oblique nematodes as well as the reproductive cycle are shown in a microscope .

The purpose of the topic . To study the structure , rotation cycle and drive efficiency of the helical - worm machine .

Short summary of the topic . Nematode It lives in the duodenum of humans . The head of the parasite is curved and has a mouth capsule . In the mouth there are sharp teeth resembling plates or very small hooks , with the help of which the parasite attaches to the mucous membrane of the intestine of its host and sucks blood .

It 's a geo g e l mint feeling . The seed was planted in the ground . With the increase in temperature , the soil has grown to about 1000 meters and has been able to stay in the soil for up to 18 months .

The work of the people is based on the crooked head of the man .The lichen is infested with dirt , and the girl 's skin is swollen and itchy .

The larvae that enter the human body are found in the small intestine . It 's all about the organization . The lychink was then moved to the back of the head . This is the year A man swallows the larvae , and the larvae fill the 12 - year - old intestine , and have sexual intercourse .

It 's not easy It feeds on its owner 's blood . In this case , the body is not satisfied with the food and water , and as a result , it becomes sick .

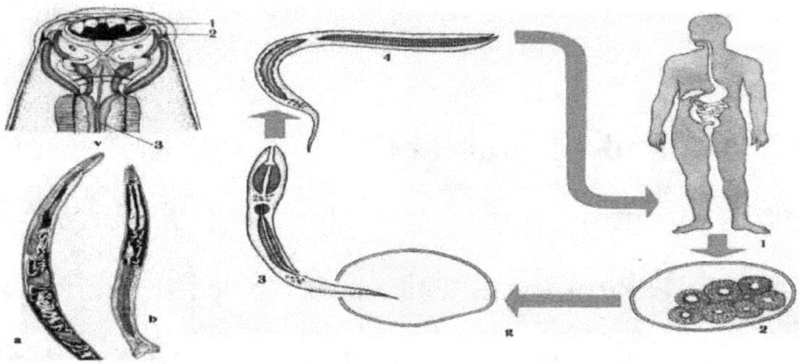

***27. Ancylostoma duodenale (Ancylostoma duodenale)** : a - **female** ; b-erk a gi; v- The mouth part of a nematode (cuticular on the oral capsule) tooth swirl) : 1 -cuticular teeth, 2-oral cavity, 3- pharynx , g- Development cycle of a roundworm : 1 -human, host of the nematode , 2 - egg, 3 -rhabditism from the egg larval emergence, 4th instar larva.*

It is recommended to be 2 years old for 5-8 years . In order to prevent this disease , first of all , it is necessary to use oblique methods . He walks on the grass , lies down on the grass , and swallows the larvae . You should not let it get to you .

Method of conducting work . Males and females are more prone to scoliosis , 5 % formalin solution . Take a look at the exterior of this chuv a lch a ng . Take one of the dirty eyes with a pair of pliers , put it in a small hole and remove it with a magnifying glass .

Control and test questions and assignments.

Draw a picture of a curved shape on a sheet of paper and write it down .

1. Nematode Which of the following organs in humans are parasites ?

2. Why is it not a crooked or twisted nematode ?
3. Nematode What is the difference between a mask and a mask ?
4. What is the length of the female and the male of the curved shape ?
5. Describe the development cycle of the roundworm nematode .
6. How many eggs does a roundworm lay in a day ?
7. How long does it take for the larva to hatch from the egg in the external environment to become infectious ?
8. How long does the larva maintain its viability in the external environment ?
9. Do you know how to bend over backwards ?

10. What is the sexual situation in the human body when the larvae are bent over the body ?

EXERCISE 10

Topic: The structure and development of the giant thornback - a representative of the phylum Echinodermata

Spiny heads (Acanthocephales) type.

Type. - Spiny-headed - **Acanthocephala**

Class -Acanthocephala

And a kil . Giant thornback ***(Macracanthorhynchus hirudinaceus)***

Echinoderms include about 500 species of parasitic worms. In adulthood, they live in the intestines of vertebrates. The anterior end of their body has become a special proboscis-like organ of attachment. The body cover consists of a thin cuticle and hypodermis. The body cavity is primary. The digestive, circulatory, and respiratory systems are absent. Echinoderms are unisexual. The excretory duct of the genital system often merges with the excretory system into a common tube. They develop by metamorphosis. The life cycle proceeds by changing hosts. This phylum includes only one class.

Class Acanthocephala. External structure. The body is hair-like, consisting of a true body and a proboscis. The inside of the proboscis is hollow, and can be turned inside out like the fingers of a glove. The loops on the wall of the proboscis, bent back, help it adhere to the intestinal wall of its host. With the help of retractor muscles, the proboscis is retracted into a special sheath. The body is covered with a thin cuticle. The hypodermis under the cuticle is formed as a result of the fusion of cells of the embryonic ectoderm. Lacunae, i.e., tubes, pass through the hypodermis. Reserve nutrients (glycogen) are accumulated in the hypodermis. On the border between the proboscis and the body, there are a pair of protrusions called *lemniscae* . The function of the lemniscae is not clear. The skin-muscle bag consists of external circular muscles and internal longitudinal muscles . Inside the muscles is a wide body cavity.

Internal structure Echinoderms are true parasites. Their digestive system is not developed. They absorb nutrients that are ready to be digested in the intestines of their host through pores on their body surface.

The reproductive organ is developed only in some species. The reproductive organ of the giant stickleback *(Macracanthorhynchus hirudinaceus)* consists of a slightly modified protonephridium. The urinary tract is fused with the genital tract. Sticklebacks are unisexual. The gonads are paired. The male has two oval testes. The vas deferens, which begin at the testes, merge to form a single oviduct. The inner part of this oviduct is covered with strong muscles and acts as a copulatory organ. This organ is located inside the oviduct sac. During mating, the sac is pulled out and covers the posterior part of the female's body. A special path of cement glands also opens into the oviduct. The secretion of the glands glues the genital opening of the fertilized female. The female reproductive system is located inside the ligament, and in young females it consists of two ovaries. During puberty, the ovaries divide into many egg fragments. These fragments break through the ligament wall and pass into the body cavity. The eggs are fertilized in the body cavity.

A single egg fragment consists of dozens of eggs. Fertilized eggs separate from the egg fragments and float in body fluids. The funnel-shaped enlarged end of the female genital tract opens into the body cavity. The next part of the genital tract forms two narrower oviducts. The eggs are sorted in the oviducts. The fertilized eggs that have passed the stage of fragmentation, from elongated hair-like, pass into the oviduct; the unfertilized, thicker eggs are released back into the body cavity. Both oviducts open into the uterus, and the uterus into the genital vagina. The genital vagina opens to the outside in the next part of the body through the genital opening. Larvae and adults of echinoderms consist of a small number of cells. In some species, the number of cells is constant.

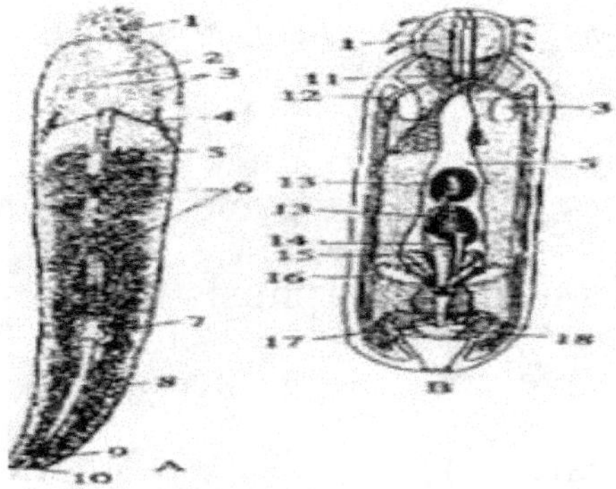

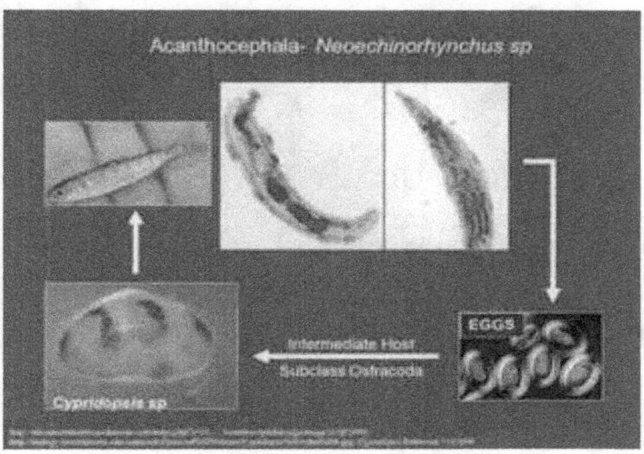

28. The structure of echinoderms. A - female. B - male: 1 - pharynx, 2 - pharynx sheath, 3 - lemnisca, 4 - vaginal muscles, 5 - ligament, 6 - ovum, 7 - cervical canal, 8 - uterus, 9 - vagina, 10 - genital opening, 11 - head ganglion, 12 - nerve trunk, 13 - testicles, 14 - seminal ducts, 15 -

cement glands, 16 - protonephridium, 17 - soot organ, 18 - soot sac .

Life cycle. The life cycle of echinoderms is associated with metamorphosis and host change. The larva develops inside the egg. When such eggs are transferred to the body of an intermediate host, larvae hatch from them. The body of the larva is elongated, with many hooks in the anterior part. For aquatic vertebrates (waterfowl, amphibians, etc.), the intermediate host is mainly small crustaceans, and for terrestrial vertebrate parasites, insects. For example, the eggs of the fish parasite Echinorhynchus salmonis develop in side-swimming fish, and the eggs of the giant echinoderm, a parasite of ants, develop in the larvae of the May beetle and the bronze beetle. The larva passes from the intestine of the intermediate host into its body cavity and sheds its hooks. The larva develops through metamorphosis and forms a young echinoderm. The young parasite has only an immature reproductive system. Its body expands, becomes spherical, and is enclosed in a thick capsule. Such a larva can survive for a long time. If the intermediate host is eaten by the primary host, the parasite emerges from the capsule in the intestine of the primary host. Its proboscis twists and sticks to the intestinal wall of the host, where it matures.

Harm. Spiny worms cause great harm to vertebrates. The giant spiny worm, which is about 25 cm long, mainly parasitizes in the intestines of pigs, damaging the intestinal wall. Pigs become infected with the parasite by eating the larvae of beetles in the soil. The spiny worm Pomphorhynchus laevis causes great harm to freshwater fish. The number of parasites in the intestines of barbel fish can reach 300. Representatives of the genus Polymorphic cause great harm to ducks; often cause mass mortality of poultry.

Phylogeny of echinoderms. There is no single general idea about the origin of echinoderms. They resemble nematodes in their cylindrical body shape, hypodermic structure, primary body cavity, and the presence of separate sexes; but they differ from them in the presence of lacunae and protonephridia in the hypodermic structure, and the structure of their reproductive system. According to another idea, echinoderms originated from priapulids. (Because the body of some priapulids is divided into a head, a smooth neck and a body covered with spines in their young stage. The excretory organ protonephridia also opens into the sexual duct, just like in echinoderms. The difference between echinoderms and priapulids is related to their parasitic lifestyle. The oldest theory about the tilogeny of echinoderms brings them closer to flatworms. The similarity of the Khartoum to the scolex of cestodes, the absence of a digestive system, the protonephridial type of the excretory system, and the presence of orthogenic characters in the nervous system indicate this. However, the structure of the adhesion organs and the disappearance of the intestine are convergent characters that arose with their parasitic lifestyle. Echinoderms should be considered as a type of animal that arose independently of flatworms and specialized in a narrow range . They are a narrow branch of the animal kingdom.

Control and test questions and assignments.

1. How many parasitic species does the echinoderm include?
2. Which animals do echinoderms parasitize in their intestines as adults?

3. How is the anterior end of the body of echinoderms structured?

4. What does the body covering of echinoderms consist of?

Main literature

1. Dadaev SD Parasitology. Textbook for students of biology majors of higher educational institutions. T., "Uzbekistan " . 2006.-207 p .

2. Dadaev S., Abdurakhmonova G. General parasitology. Textbook for master's degree students of higher educational institutions specializing in biology. T., "Science and Technology". 2013.-384 p.

3. Dadayev S. Laboratory exercises in parasitology. Methodological guide for students of biology majors in higher education institutions. Gulistan, 2019 y .

4. Dadaev S., Dadaeva D.S. Laboratory practice of parasitology. Methodological method Tashkent, 2019

Additional literature

1. Dadaev S.D., Solodovnikova O.G. Parasitology. Uchebnoe posobie. Tashkent, 2021. 221 p

2. Abdurakhmanova G., Dadyev S. Practical exercises in general parasitology. Textbook for master's degree students of higher educational institutions specializing in biology (zoology). Tashkent. 2020, 282 p .

3. Dogel V.A. Obshaya parasitology. - Leningrad. 1962. -464 c

4. Ginetsinskaya T.A., Dobrovolsky A.A. Chastnaya parasitology. Uchebnoe posobie, t.1. M., 1978.

5. Ginetsinskaya T.A., Dobrovolsky A.A. Chastnaya parasitology. Uchebnoe posobie, t.1. M., 1978.

6. B. Kholiknazarov. Zoology (systematics, genetic and evolutionary aspects). Tashkent 2023

7. Korotova D.M. i dr. Parasitology and invasive animal diseases: method. instructions for laboratory work for special purpose 36.05.01 Veterinarii. "Saratovsky GAU".- Saratov, 2015.- 242 p.

Electronic information sources :

www.pedagog.uz

www.edu.uz

www.natlib.uz (Uzbek National Library named after A. Navoi)

http://ziyonet.uz — Ziyonet information and educational resources portal